P9-DTQ-672

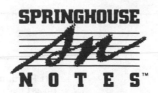

SPRINGHOUSE

NOTES™

# PERIOPERATIVE NURSING

**Linda B. Chitwood, RN, MSN, CRNA**
Ms. Chitwood, coauthor of this book, is a nurse anesthetist (certified by the American Association of Nurse Anesthetists) in private practice in Memphis, Tennessee. She received her BSN from Memphis State University and her MSN from Rush University, Chicago. Ms. Chitwood is a member of the American Medical Writers Association and the American Marketing Association. She is also president of Media Medical, Inc., Memphis.

**Diane Crisler Swain, RN, BSN, CNOR**
Ms. Swain, coauthor of this book, is the director of Le Bonheur East Surgery Center, Memphis, Tennessee, and previously served as clinical instructor for intraoperative nursing at the Methodist Hospital School of Nursing, Memphis. She received her BSN from the University of Tennessee, Memphis, and her certification in operating room nursing from the Association of Operating Room Nurses. Ms. Swain is a member of the Association of Operating Room Nurses.

**Barbara Kascsak Bailes, RN, EdD**
Dr. Bailes, reviewer of this book, is an Assistant Professor of Nursing at the University of Texas Health Science Center at Houston School of Nursing. She received her BSN from Incarnate Word College, San Antonio, Texas; her MS from Texas Women's University, Houston, and her EdD from the University of Houston. Dr. Bailes is a member of the National League for Nursing, the Association of Operating Room Nurses, and Sigma Theta Tau.

Springhouse Corporation
Springhouse, Pennsylvania

# Staff

**Executive Director, Editorial**
Stanley Loeb

**Director of Trade and Textbooks**
Minnie B. Rose, RN, BSN, MEd

**Art Director**
John Hubbard

**Clinical Consultant**
Maryann Foley, RN, BSN

**Editor**
David Moreau

**Copy Editor**
Mary Hohenhaus Hardy

**Designers**
Stephanie Peters (associate art director),
Jacalyn Facciolo

**Art Production**
Robert Perry (manager), Anna Brindisi, Donald
Knauss, Tom Robbins, Robert Wieder

**Typography**
David Kosten (director), Diane Paluba (manager),
Elizabeth Bergman, Joyce Rossi Biletz, Phyllis
Marron, Robin Rantz, Valerie L. Rosenberger

**Manufacturing**
Deborah Meiris (manager), T.A. Landis,
Jennifer Suter

The author and the publisher disclaim responsibility for any
adverse effects resulting directly or indirectly from any sug-
gested procedures herein, from any undetected errors, or
from the reader's misunderstanding of the text.

© 1992 by Springhouse Corporation, 1111 Bethlehem Pike,
Springhouse, PA 19477. All rights reserved. Reproduction in
whole or part by any means whatsoever without written permission of the publisher is prohibited by law. Authorization to
photocopy any items for internal or personal use, or the internal or personal use of specific clients, is granted by Springhouse Corporation for users registered with the Copyright
Clearance Center (CCC) Transactional Reporting Service,
provided that the base fee of $00.00 per copy plus $.75 per
page is paid directly to CCC, 27 Congress St., Salem, MA
01970. For those organizations that have been granted a license by CCC, a separate system of payment has been ar-
ranged. The fee code for users of the Transactional Reporting
Service is 0874343682/92 $00.00 + $.75.
Printed in the United States of America.

SN18-010791

Library of Congress Cataloging-in-Publication Data

Chitwood, Linda B.
  Perioperative nursing / Linda B. Chitwood,
Diane Crisler Swain [coauthors]; Barbara
Kascsak Bailes [reviewer].
    p. cm. — (Springhouse notes)
  Includes bibliographical references and index.
  1. Operating room nursing—Outlines, syllabi,
etc. I. Swain, Diane Crisler. II. Bailes, Barbara
Kascsak. III. Title. IV. Series.
  [DNLM: 1. Operating Room Nursing—outlines.
  WY 18 C543p]
RD32.3.C45    1992
610.73′677—dc20
DNLM/DLC                              91-4737
ISBN 0-87434-368-2                         CIP

# Contents

# How to Use Springhouse Notes

Today, more than ever, nursing students face enormous time pressures. Nursing education has become more sophisticated, increasing the difficulties students have with studying efficiently and keeping pace.

The need for a comprehensive, well-designed series of study aids is great, which is why we've produced Springhouse Notes...to meet that need. Springhouse Notes provide essential course material in outline form, enabling the nursing student to study more effectively, improve understanding, achieve higher test scores, and get better grades.

Key features appear throughout each book, making the information more accessible and easier to remember.
- **Learning Objectives.** These objectives precede each section in the book to help the student evaluate knowledge before and after study.
- **Key Points.** Highlighted throughout the book, these points provide a way to quickly review critical information. Key points may include:
  - a cardinal sign or symptom of a disorder
  - the most current or popular theory about a topic
  - a distinguishing characteristic of a disorder
  - the most important step of a process
  - a critical assessment component
  - a crucial nursing intervention
  - the most widely used or successful therapy or treatment.
- **Points to Remember.** This information, found at the end of each section, summarizes the section in capsule form.
- **Glossary.** Difficult, frequently used, or sometimes misunderstood terms are defined for the student at the end of each section.

**Remember:** Springhouse Notes are learning tools designed to *help* you. They are not intended for use as a primary information source. They should never substitute for class attendance, text reading, or classroom note-taking.

This book, *Perioperative Nursing,* presents concepts essential to each phase of surgical intervention. Important topics include preoperative and postoperative assessment and teaching, preanesthesia evaluation, anesthesia types and anesthetic agents, surgical suite design and traffic flow, instrumentation, patient positioning, intraoperative complications, infection control, ambulatory surgery, and legal considerations.

# Overview of Perioperative Nursing

**Learning Objectives**

After studying this section, the reader should be able to:

- Define perioperative nursing practice.

- Describe specific responsibilities of perioperative nurses.

- List the three major classifications of surgery.

- Identify the three phases of the perioperative period.

## I. Overview of Perioperative Nursing

### A. Introduction

1. Perioperative nursing is the comprehensive nursing care of a patient before, during, and after surgery
2. The perioperative period begins with the decision for surgery and ends when surgery-related nursing care is no longer required
3. Perioperative nursing has become a specialty
   a. The Association of Operating Room Nurses (AORN) was founded in 1949
   b. In 1978, the AORN defined the perioperative role of the operating room nurse as those activities performed during the preoperative, intraoperative, and postoperative phases
   c. Perioperative nursing practice is guided by the AORN's *Standards and Recommended Practices for Perioperative Nursing,* developed in collaboration with the American Nurses Association and first published in 1981
4. Perioperative nurses are responsible for:
   a. Providing care for the patient during a period of forced dependency, when anesthesia-induced loss of normal physiologic responses places the patient at high risk for injuries
   b. Ensuring continuity of care by coordinating the activities of other surgical team members and documenting the events that occur
   c. Keeping abreast of constantly changing technology
   d. Incorporating knowledge of the classifications of surgery into the plan of care

### B. Classifications of surgery

1. General information
   a. Perioperative nursing revolves around surgery — the treatment of an illness or injury by invasive means
   b. Surgery imposes physical and mental stressors on the patient
   c. Surgery places the patient at risk for injury because of the inherent danger of most procedures and because anesthesia produces loss of sensation and protective reflexes
   d. Surgery is classified according to degree of urgency, degree of risk, or purpose (or a combination of these)
2. Degree of urgency
   a. Refers to the time available to the patient, the family, and the health care team to decide whether or not surgery will be performed
   b. Usually corresponds to the severity of the patient's injury or illness
   c. May be categorized as *elective* (scheduled in advance, based on the patient's health), *urgent* (usually performed within 48 hours of deciding that surgery is needed), or *emergency* (must be performed immediately to save the patient's life or to avoid life-threatening complications)

3. Degree of risk
   a. Refers to the relative threat that surgery poses to the patient
   b. May be categorized as *major* (may pose a great threat to the patient, usually requires hospitalization, is a prolonged procedure, involves major body organs, and carries considerable potential for complications) or *minor* (poses a minimal threat to the patient, usually takes place in a physician's office or clinic, is a brief procedure, and has few complications)
4. Purpose
   a. Surgery is performed for diagnostic, ablative, palliative, reconstructive, transplantation, or constructive purposes
   b. Diagnostic surgery helps a physician make or confirm a diagnosis
   c. Ablative surgery removes a diseased or injured body part
   d. Palliative surgery relieves or decreases the intensity of an illness or injury but does not cure it
   e. Reconstructive surgery rebuilds or restores function to an injured or damaged area
   f. Transplantation surgery removes damaged organs or tissues and replaces them with functioning ones
   g. Constructive surgery reestablishes the function of a body part that is congenitally malformed

## C. Phases of the perioperative period
1. General information
   a. The three phases of the perioperative period are preoperative, intraoperative, and postoperative
   b. In large institutions, the perioperative nursing staff usually consists of a preoperative nurse, an intraoperative nurse, and a postoperative nurse
   c. In smaller institutions, the perioperative nurse may provide all nursing care for a surgical patient
   d. Clear communication through documentation and reporting is essential when more than one person provides perioperative nursing care
2. Preoperative phase
   a. Begins with the decision for surgery and ends when the patient is transferred to the operating room
   b. Aims to prepare the patient for surgery; typical activities include preoperative patient teaching, skin preparation, and medication administration
3. Intraoperative phase
   a. Begins when the patient is placed on the operating room bed and ends when he is transferred to the postanesthesia care unit (PACU)
   b. Aims to protect the patient during surgery; typical activities include surgical asepsis and minimizing traffic flow

4. Postoperative phase
   a. Begins when the patient is admitted to the PACU and ends when surgery-related nursing care is no longer required
   b. Aims to alleviate the patient's pain and nausea and support the patient until normal physiologic responses return; typical activities include medication administration, monitoring fluid intake and output and respiratory and cardiovascular functioning

## Points to Remember

Surgical patients, especially those undergoing major surgery, are at risk for injury because of the inherent danger of most procedures and because anesthesia produces loss of sensation and protective reflexes.

Surgery is classified according to degree of urgency, degree of risk, or purpose (or a combination of these).

The perioperative period includes preoperative, intraoperative, and postoperative phases.

Detailed documentation and reporting of perioperative events help ensure clear communication among staff and facilitate continuity of care for the patient.

## Glossary

**Continuity of care** — uninterrupted patient care, especially when responsibility for care changes from person to person

**Standards of nursing practice** — written guidelines for providing patient care and criteria for evaluating that care

**Surgery**   invasive procedure used to correct deformities, repair injuries, and treat, diagnose, or remove diseased tissues

# Perioperative Team

**Learning Objectives**

After studying this section, the reader should be able to:

● Define perioperative team.

● Identify all perioperative team members and describe their functions.

## II. Perioperative Team

### A. Introduction
1. The perioperative team consists of individuals involved in patient care during one or more phases of surgery
2. Members of the perioperative team include:
   a. Preoperative nurse
   b. Surgeon
   c. Anesthetist
   d. Scrub nurse
   e. Circulating nurse
   f. Surgical assistant
   g. Postanesthesia care unit (PACU) nurse
   h. Postoperative nurse
3. Each team member has specific functions, some of which overlap to ensure continuity of care
4. Clear communication among team members and coordination of their activities improve the chances of a favorable outcome

### B. Preoperative nurse
1. General information
   a. A preoperative nurse is usually a registered nurse (RN) but can be a licensed practical nurse (LPN) working under the supervision of an RN
   b. A preoperative nurse must know the patient's physical condition and pertinent history and the planned treatment
2. Functions
   a. Prepares the patient physically and emotionally for surgery
   b. Collects and analyzes data that may affect care given by surgical and postsurgical team members
   c. Completes the preoperative checklist and ensures that all necessary data are recorded on the chart

### C. Surgeon
1. General information
   a. A surgeon has completed a residency program approved by the American Board of Surgery and may or may not be board certified
   b. A board-certified surgeon has successfully completed a certifying examination in a surgical specialty
2. Functions
   a. Identifies the need for surgery and, with the patient and other specialists, determines and plans appropriate treatment
   b. Discusses surgical risks, benefits, possible complications, and treatment alternatives with the patient
   c. Obtains informed consent and performs the operation
   d. Provides postoperative medical care, as indicated

**D. Anesthetist**
1. General information
   a. An anesthetist may be a physician who is or is not certified by the American Board of Anesthesia
   b. An anesthetist may be a certified registered nurse anesthetist (CRNA) — an RN with critical care experience who has completed an accredited program of nurse anesthesia and has passed a certifying examination
2. Functions
   a. Assesses the patient and determines the type of anesthetic agent to be administered
   b. Discusses the type of anesthetic and its benefits, possible risks, complications, and alternative choices with the patient
   c. Obtains informed consent for anesthesia and administers the anesthetic
   d. Provides pain relief and relaxation during the perioperative period by administering additional agents, such as analgesics and muscle relaxants
   e. Maintains airway control and gas exchange during surgery with endotracheal tubes, masks, and ventilation devices
   f. Monitors the patient's physiologic status during surgery and intervenes when necessary
   g. Evaluates the patient's postoperative response to the anesthesia and discharges the patient from the PACU

**E. Scrub nurse**
1. General information
   a. A scrub nurse may be an RN or a certified surgical technologist (CST)
   b. A scrub nurse must have appropriate knowledge of the surgical instruments and suture materials to be used
   c. A scrub nurse works primarily with sterile instruments and equipment
2. Functions
   a. Creates a sterile field by opening a large sterile pack of towels and drapes onto an empty table and then placing sterile supplies and instruments onto it
   b. Arranges instruments, drapes, and sutures on the back table and Mayo stand for easy retrieval
   c. Passes instruments and sutures to the surgeon at the appropriate time, enabling the surgeon to operate without interruption
   d. Counts instruments, needles, and sponges with the circulating nurse before the incision, before wound closure, and after the procedure to ensure that all surgical equipment has been removed from the patient
   e. Maintains sterility of instruments until the patient is transferred to the PACU so that the wound can be reexplored immediately if excessive bleeding occurs
   f. Prepares instruments and equipment for transport to the decontamination area after the patient has been taken to the PACU

**F. Circulating nurse**
1. General information
   a. A circulating nurse is an RN who has completed 6 months to 1 year of operating room orientation and has acquired the skills necessary to provide direct patient care during surgery
   b. A circulating nurse must have appropriate knowledge of anatomy, physiology, and pathophysiology
2. Functions
   a. Assembles necessary equipment and supplies for the procedure
   b. Conducts a preoperative nursing assessment of the patient
   c. Establishes rapport with the patient and family members in the preoperative holding area and provides emotional support by addressing concerns and explaining operating room events
   d. Ensures patient safety intraoperatively by preventing injury from incorrect body positioning, hazardous equipment, hypothermia, retention of foreign bodies, blood loss, and infection
   e. Documents events on the operating room clinical record

**G. Surgical assistant**
1. General information
   a. A surgical assistant may be a surgeon, resident, intern, medical student, RN, or CST
   b. A surgical assistant must have sufficient knowledge, skill, and experience to properly and adequately assist the surgeon and act for the benefit of the patient
2. Functions
   a. Exposes the surgical site to the surgeon by retracting tissue and removing blood and fluids
   b. Assists in maintaining patient hemostasis using cautery, suture ties, and clips
   c. Assists with wound closure by approximating wound edges with suture materials or clips and applying a surgical dressing

**H. PACU nurse**
1. General information
   a. A PACU nurse is an RN experienced in postanesthesia recovery care
   b. A PACU nurse must have appropriate monitoring ability and knowledge of anesthetic and reversal agents
2. Functions
   a. Obtains anesthetist's report on the type of anesthetic administered, the patient's general condition, and any significant preoperative history or intraoperative events
   b. Maintains a patent airway until the patient recovers from the anesthetic, monitors the patient's vital signs and general condition, and remains alert for signs of bleeding
   c. Administers antiemetic and pain medications, as indicated

    d. Evaluates the patient to determine readiness for discharge from the PACU and reports patient status to the anesthetist

    e. Accompanies the patient to the nursing unit and reports patient's condition to the receiving nurse

    f. Obtains vital signs after the patient has been transferred to a bed to ensure patient's stability before admission to a unit

## I. Postoperative nurse

1. General information

    a. A postoperative nurse is usually an RN but can be an LPN working under the supervision of an RN

    b. A postoperative nurse must have knowledge of preoperative and intraoperative events

2. Functions

    a. Communicates with and receives report from the PACU nurse regarding intraoperative events and the patient's status

    b. Assesses the patient's overall condition on arrival from the PACU and while in the nursing unit

    c. Monitors the patient's vital signs, level of consciousness, cardiac and respiratory status, and gastrointestinal and urinary functions

    d. Facilitates the patient's return to an optimal level of functioning by encouraging early ambulation and self-care

    e. Provides postoperative teaching and prepares the patient for discharge from the hospital

    f. Arranges for follow-up services as necessary

## Points to Remember

The perioperative team consists of the preoperative nurse, surgeon, anesthetist, scrub nurse, circulating nurse, surgical assistant, PACU nurse, and postoperative nurse.

Coordination of all team member activities improves the chances of a favorable outcome.

Anesthesia can be administered by a physician or a CRNA.

The scrub nurse works primarily with sterile instruments and equipment.

## Glossary

**Anesthetist** — person prepared to administer anesthesia

**Certified surgical technologist (CST)** — person who has completed a 1- to 2-year program on the technical aspects of operating room nursing and has successfully passed a certifying examination

**Hemostasis** — control or arrest of bleeding

**Informed consent** — permission given by the patient for the surgeon to perform the operation, provided that the patient understands the purpose of the surgery and its risks, benefits, possible complications, and alternatives

**Mayo stand** — frame with a removable rectangular instrument tray that is placed above and across the patient below the operation site; the base of the stand slides under the operating table

**Preoperative checklist** — form used by health-care team members to document actions that the facility requires before the patient is taken to the operating room

# Perioperative Infection Control

**Learning Objectives**

After studying this section, the reader should be able to:

- Define aseptic technique.

- Describe the patient's and team members' skin preparation.

- Discuss creation and maintenance of the sterile field.

- Identify two sterilization methods.

- Describe two types of steam autoclaves.

- Identify three chemicals used for sterilization.

- Describe two methods for monitoring sterilization effectiveness.

- Discuss precautions that protect against infectious diseases.

## III. Perioperative Infection Control

### A. Introduction

1. During the perioperative period, the risk of infection is high for the patient (because the first line of defense against infection — intact skin — is breached) and for the team members (through contact with blood and other body fluids)
2. Precautions are necessary to protect the patient and team members from potential infectious agents
3. Perioperative team members must use caution when caring for surgical patients, all of whom should be considered potentially infectious

### B. Patient protection

1. General information
   a. *Aseptic technique* incorporates principles and practices developed to create and maintain an environment free from infectious agents; this technique is used with all surgical procedures
   b. Items that come into contact with the surgical wound must be sterile
   c. When a sterile item touches an unsterile item or substance, contamination occurs and the risk of infection increases
   d. If an item cannot be made sterile, it is rendered *surgically clean* by mechanical washing and disinfection, which destroys many, but not all, microorganisms
2. Preparing the team members' skin
   a. Because the skin cannot be made sterile, it is washed with an antimicrobial scrub solution and covered with sterile barriers
   b. Surgical team members conduct a regimented handscrub beginning with the four sides of each finger from thumb to fifth finger and continuing over the back of the hand, the palm, the wrist, and up the arm to approximately two inches above the elbow
   c. The *counted stroke* handscrub method uses a specified number of strokes for each area, usually 30 strokes for the nails and 20 strokes for each of the skin areas
   d. The *timed scrub* procedure uses a specified amount of time for scrubbing each area; each nail is scrubbed for 30 seconds then repeated once more; the hands and arms to the elbow are scrubbed for 3 minutes each
   c. After completing the regimented handscrub, the team member holds the arms and hands upright with the elbows flexed to prevent contamination of scrubbed areas by unscrubbed areas, while being assisted in donning sterile gowns and gloves
3. Preparing the patient's skin
   a. The preoperative nurse prepares the patient's skin by thoroughly washing it with an antimicrobial soap or detergent (pHisoDerm, Hibiclens, or Betadine) and sometimes clipping or shaving the patient's hair, if ordered

    b. The circulating nurse performs a final scrub, starting at the proposed incision site and scrubbing for a specified amount of time with sterile sponges, proceeding in a circular motion to the periphery, discarding the sponge, and beginning again with a clean sponge

    c. The scrub proceeds from areas considered clean to those considered unclean; areas known to contain large amounts of bacteria, such as open wounds or body orifices, are prepared last

4. Creating the sterile field
    a. The sterile field, an area of asepsis created by unwrapping a large sterile pack onto a table, is created as near to the time of surgery as possible and always monitored to avoid contamination
    b. All items used within a sterile field are sterile
    c. Packages of sterile items are inspected for possible perforation, permeation by liquid, and outdated sterilization dates, indicating that the item is no longer sterile and should not be used
    d. Sterile items added to the sterile field must not touch unsterile areas, such as the hands of the person opening the package or the edges of wrappers and packages
    e. The patient becomes the center of the sterile field through placement of sterile drapes (towels, sheets, and plastic materials) that protect the surgical site from contamination and establish a work area for the surgical team

5. Maintaining the sterile field
    a. The sterile field encompasses the sterile table containing the items necessary for the procedure, the draped patient, and team members wearing sterile gowns
    b. The front of the surgical gown from chest to table level and the sleeves from above the elbow to the cuff are considered sterile; the back of the gown, neckline, under the arms, and the gown below table level are considered unsterile
    c. Gowns or gloves that tear or become permeated by solutions must be immediately replaced or reinforced
    d. Team members approach the sterile field face first to maintain asepsis and prevent contamination; movement around the sterile field should be limited to avoid compromising sterility
    e. Sterile team members remain near the sterile field — and unsterile personnel remain away from it — to avoid accidental contamination
    f. Sterile team members should pass each other face to face (sterile to sterile) or back to back (unsterile to unsterile)
    g. When solutions are added to the sterile field on the table, the scrub nurse places the receptacle near the edge of the table so that the circulating nurse can pour the solution without reaching across the sterile field

6. Nursing responsibilities
    a. Preserve the patient's privacy and dignity
    b. Take measures to prevent heat loss during skin preparation

    c. Maintain constant attention to the sterile field: carefully examine the packages of all sterile items before opening any of them, and address and correct all breaks in aseptic technique immediately

    d. Keep doors of the operating room closed when creating the sterile field and during surgery, except when team members are entering or leaving, to prevent airborne contamination

    e. Do not allow team members with draining skin lesions or upper respiratory tract infections to be involved in direct patient care until the employee health department or team member's physician provides written permission

**C. Sterilization**

  1. General information

    a. Sterilization destroys all microorganisms, including spores, without damaging surgical items and without leaving toxic residues that could harm human tissue

    b. Sterilization is accomplished most commonly with steam or with chemicals

  2. Steam sterilization

    a. Uses heat and moisture under pressure in an autoclave; the heated moisture must come in contact with the entire surface of the item being sterilized

    b. Is relatively inexpensive and can sterilize most items used in the operating room

    c. Destroys microorganisms by denaturing and coagulating cell protein

    d. Is accomplished at temperatures ranging from 250° to 270° F (121° to 132° C) and at pressures of 15 to 27 psi

    e. Requires air (which is heavier than steam) to be removed from the autoclave for total contact to occur

    f. Requires varying amounts of time, depending on size and shape of the item, type of autoclave used, temperature setting, and whether the item is wrapped

  3. Autoclaves

    a. Autoclaves can be gravity-displaced or high-vacuum

    b. In gravity-displacement autoclaves, steam enters the chamber from the top and air is pushed out the bottom

    c. Most flash autoclaves are gravity-displacement machines used to quickly sterilize unwrapped instruments before and during surgery

    d. High-vacuum autoclaves use a vacuum pump to remove air before injecting steam, which enables steam contact with large, packaged items (such as wrapped instrument trays and packs) within moments

  4. Chemical sterilization

    a. Uses toxic gas or liquid chemicals to sterilize items that cannot withstand the heat and pressure of steam sterilization

    b. Destroys microorganisms by inactivating the reproductive abilities of the cells

    c. Is more expensive and time consuming than steam sterilization

    d. Requires items to be dry to permit contact with all surface areas and prevent dilution of the sterilizing agent

5. Types of chemicals

    a. The most commonly used gas is ethylene oxide, which is highly flammable, explosive, and toxic

    b. Ethylene oxide sterilization is affected by the concentration of gas, temperature, humidity, and ability of gas to penetrate the wrapper

    c. Because the gas is toxic, items must be mechanically aerated (the preferred method requires a minimum of four air exchanges per hour for 8 to 12 hours) or ambiently aerated (requires 1 to 7 days, depending on the type of material used)

    d. Formaldehyde, a liquid chemical, is rarely used as a sterilizing agent because of its odor and the length of time required for sterilization (12 to 24 hours)

    e. Glutaraldehyde 2%, also a liquid, can sterilize items in 10 hours, is less irritating than formaldehyde, and is commonly used as a high-level disinfecting agent

    f. High-level disinfection of instruments is accomplished by soaking items for 10 minutes in glutaraldehyde 2%

6. Assurance of sterility

    a. Chemical indicators—tape or strips placed on the outside and the inside of the package—change color during steam sterilization; they are used as screening devices to determine if an item has been sterilized but do not ensure sterilization

    b. Biologic monitoring, the most effective method of testing sterilization, uses commercially manufactured strips, ampules, or capsules containing known spore-forming organisms

    c. Once subjected to sterilization, these biologic indicators are incubated and tested for growth, with a positive test indicating that conditions necessary for sterilization have not been met

7. Nursing responsibilities

    a. Prepare items to be sterilized by ensuring that they are clean and free from residue

    b. Dry items to be chemically sterilized and avoid direct contact with chemicals

    c. Open the lumens of tubing and position items undergoing steam sterilization to ensure that the steam can contact all surface areas

    d. Check the autoclave charts indicating the temperature reached and the time of sterilization with each load

    e. Examine the chemical indicators on the outside of the wrapper before placing the item on the sterile field

    f. Rinse chemically sterilized items thoroughly with sterile water before use to prevent tissue injury

## D. Team members' protection

1. General information
   a. All items coming in contact with a patient's blood or other body fluids are considered contaminated, and perioperative team members must adhere to universal blood and body fluid precautions
   b. Cuts or sticks from contaminated instruments or needles and exposure to mucous membranes should be reported immediately to the employee health department for follow-up evaluation and treatment

2. Barriers
   a. Masks, glasses or goggles, gloves, and gowns are barriers that protect team members from blood during surgery
   b. Masks and glasses or goggles protect the eyes and face and should be worn by all sterile team members and persons conducting or assisting with intubation
   c. Gloves and gowns protect the hands and arms and should be worn by all sterile team members, persons starting I.V. or arterial lines, and those handling objects contaminated with blood
   d. Persons with cuts or rashes on the hands or arms should wear gloves and gowns at all times in the operating room, even if not in direct patient contact

3. Preoperative protection
   a. Wash hands before entering the patient's room or operating room and before and after any patient contact
   b. Clean all equipment, flat surfaces, and surgical lights with a disinfectant solution before each surgical procedure
   c. Don appropriate barriers before patient contact

4. Intraoperative protection
   a. Minimize contact with any part of the operating room table that becomes contaminated with blood or other body fluids
   b. Discard disposable items that touch contaminated fluids in plastic bags, and dispose of sharp items in impervious containers
   c. Handle sharp items with extreme caution to avoid being stuck, and do not recap needles
   d. Use a disinfecting solution to clean areas that become contaminated with blood and other body fluids
   e. Use gloves to handle specimens, and immediately change scrub suits contaminated with blood

5. Postoperative protection
   a. Wear gloves during extubation, dressing changes, insertion of I.V. tubes, and withdrawal of blood
   b. Change gloves and wash hands between patient contacts
   c. Wear masks and goggles during extubation and suctioning when splashing is possible

6. Nursing responsibilities
   a. Exercise caution when handling sharp items contaminated by blood and body fluids
   b. Monitor other team members for compliance with universal blood and body fluid precautions
   c. Clean blood spills immediately with disinfecting solutions, and report all significant exposures to nursing supervisors

## Points to Remember

The hands and arms of scrubbed team members are surgically clean but not sterile.

Sterile fields must be constantly monitored and kept in view.

Contamination occurs whenever sterile barriers are violated.

Packaging of sterile items must be carefully checked before placing any item on the sterile field.

Items must be clean before undergoing sterilization.

Because the sterilizing agent must come in contact with all surface areas of the item to be sterilized, proper preparation and positioning are necessary.

All surgical patients are potentially infectious.

Surgical team members are at high risk for infections transmitted by blood and other body fluids.

## Glossary

**Autoclave** — two-chambered apparatus that can sterilize items with pressurized steam

**Denaturation** — changing chemical composition of a substance, resulting in loss of some or all of its characteristics

**Disinfectant** — chemical agent that kills pathogenic organisms but may be ineffective against spores

**Spore** — reproductive element of some types of bacteria that is resistant to most disinfecting techniques and difficult to kill

**Sterile** — free from all living organisms, including spores

**Universal blood and body fluid precautions** — guidelines established by the Centers for Disease Control that outline steps to take when exposed to blood and other body fluids, based on the premise that all patients are potentially infectious

# Preoperative Nursing

**Learning Objectives**
After studying this section, the reader should be able to:

● Identify components of the preoperative nursing assessment.

● Identify components of the preoperative teaching plan.

● Describe how a patient is prepared for surgery.

● Discuss major responsibilities of the preoperative nurse.

● Explain the purpose of a preanesthesia evaluation.

● Name the five classifications of a patient's physical status and describe their significance.

## IV. Preoperative Nursing

### A. Introduction

1. The preoperative phase begins when the patient decides to have surgery and consists primarily of collecting and analyzing data used to help plan intraoperative events
2. The nurse's primary responsibility is to prepare the patient physically and emotionally for surgery (see Appendix A, Nursing Process Applied to the Preoperative Phase)
3. Accurate and thorough documentation and clear communication are essential to ensure continuity of patient care

### B. Nursing assessment

1. General information
   a. A comprehensive nursing assessment, consisting of a nursing history, physical examination, and patient identification immediately before surgery, enables the nursing staff to provide individualized patient care
   b. A well-documented preoperative assessment provides the intraoperative and postoperative team members with essential baseline information that cannot be obtained from an unconscious or sedated patient
2. Nursing history
   a. Chief complaint or reason for the visit, documented mostly in the patient's own words
   b. Existing and past medical problems, injuries, and surgery
   c. Food and drug allergies, including reactions described in the patient's own words
   d. Current medications, prescription and nonprescription
   e. Smoking history, including number of pack-years smoked
   f. Mobility impairment
   g. Communication limitations, such as language barriers or illiteracy
   h. Psychosocial aspects, such as the patient's perception of the surgery and the availability of emotional support
3. Physical examination
   a. General condition—vital signs and temperature
   b. Head and neck—condition of oral mucous membranes, presence of jugular vein distention
   c. Skin—general condition; turgor; rashes, abrasions, discoloration, or pustules; condition of planned surgical site
   d. Thorax and lungs—normal or abnormal breath sounds, rate and character of respirations, use of accessory muscles for breathing, use of pillows or supports
   e. Cardiovascular status—heart sounds, apical and peripheral pulses, blood pressure
   f. Abdomen—bowel sounds; shape, size, and symmetry; distention or scars
   g. Neurologic status—level of consciousness, motor and sensory function, neurologic deficits

4. Patient identification
   a. Is documented in the clinical record to avoid inadvertently performing the wrong surgical procedure on the patient
   b. Verifies the patient's and surgeon's names, proposed surgical procedure, and anatomic site of the procedure as stated by the patient and correlates this information with the operating room schedule, medical record, and patient identification bracelet
   c. Requires nonresponsive patients to be identified by the surgeon
5. Nursing responsibilities
   a. Notify the surgeon of long-term aspirin use, use of anticoagulants or steroids, infection at or near the surgical site, and elevated temperature that could affect the outcome of surgery
   b. Document the nursing assessment and verify patient identification, informing the surgeon of any discrepancies
   c. Alert the postanesthesia care unit (PACU) staff of conditions — such as neurologic deficits, absent or diminished peripheral pulses, or breathing difficulties — that could affect postoperative assessment or care

## C. Preoperative teaching
1. General information
   a. Information provided by the nurse may help alleviate the patient's fear and anxiety before surgery
   b. Teaching plans must be individualized because people learn at different rates and through different teaching methods
   c. A *learning assessment* — evaluation of a patient's knowledge of his condition, perception of surgery, and cultural background — provides baseline data for developing a preoperative teaching plan
2. Teaching methods
   a. Discussion
   b. Demonstration
   c. Written instructions and pamphlets
   d. Visual aids (videotapes, drawings, slides, and charts)
3. Teaching plan content
   a. Review the procedure — its purpose, anticipated duration, and expected postoperative course
   b. Explain preoperative events — diagnostic tests, skin preparation, I.V. insertion, sedation, and transfer to the holding area
   c. Explain intraoperative events — function of the circulating nurse, application of monitoring equipment, administration of anesthesia, maintenance of privacy and dignity, staff communication with family members during the procedure, and transport to the PACU
   d. Explain postoperative events — expected length of stay in the PACU; effective coughing, deep breathing, and turning; presence of indwelling catheters or drains; nursing support; pain control; and need for early ambulation

4. Nursing responsibilities
   a. Include family members or significant others in the teaching plan to alleviate the patient's anxiety and to reinforce information given to the patient
   b. Motivate the patient to learn by providing relevant information
   c. Obtain feedback or demonstration from the patient to determine the effectiveness of teaching methods
   d. Document the teaching plan and the patient's response, preferably in the patient's own words

**D. Preoperative preparation**
   1. General information
      a. Preoperative preparation ensures that the patient is in optimal physical condition before surgery
      b. Preoperative preparation ensures that the patient understands perioperative events and receives emotional support from the nursing staff and family members
   2. Preoperative orders
      a. Food and fluids are usually withheld 6 to 8 hours before surgery to decrease gastric contents; noncompliance with nothing-by-mouth (NPO) orders may necessitate cancellation of elective surgery because of the markedly increased risk of gastroesophageal reflux aspiration, which can result in aspiration pneumonitis, respiratory arrest, or death
      b. Patient skin preparation usually includes a bath the night before surgery and, just before surgery, removal of hair at the surgical site, using a depilatory, electric clippers, or sterile razor; heads of clippers are disinfected carefully between each use to prevent colonization of microorganisms in nicked areas, which can cause postoperative infections
      c. Before gastrointestinal procedures, enemas and cathartics are usually given to expel bowel contents, providing easier access to the surgical site and preventing contents from spilling into the peritoneal cavity, which could cause infection
      d. Urinary catheterization is usually ordered for pelvic procedures (to decompress the bladder, providing better access to the surgical site and decreasing the possibility of inadvertent bladder laceration) or for any lengthy procedure (to drain the bladder and monitor urine output)
      e. Hemoglobin, hematocrit, and chemistry profiles are needed for a patient undergoing general anesthesia, and blood type and crossmatching are performed before any procedure with a potential for excessive blood loss
      f. A sickle cell test is ordered for black patients to rule out sickle cell anemia, which would adversely affect the surgical outcome
      g. An electrocardiogram (ECG) and chest X-ray are ordered if indicated by the patient's history, such as pulmonary or cardiac problems
      h. An I.V. line is inserted for fluid replacement and drug administration (see *Using a preoperative checklist,* page 28)

## USING A PREOPERATIVE CHECKLIST

Before a patient leaves the nursing unit for surgery, all preoperative procedures must be completed. The nurse can use a checklist like the one shown below to avoid overlooking important details. As each procedure is completed, the nurse or other health care professional responsible for the procedure checks it off and initials the list. An operating room nurse in the holding area double-checks each item on the checklist before the patient enters the operating room.

Patient's name _Marian Welsch_

Room _403ᴬ_      Date _7/21/91_

| | | | |
|---|---|---|---|
| ID band | ✓ | | LK JD |
| History and physical | ✓ | | LK |
| Physicians' consultations | ✓ | | LK |
| Consent form | ✓ | | LK |
| Blood type and crossmatch | ✓ | | LK |
| Complete blood count | ✓ | | LK |
| Urinalysis | ✓ | | LK |
| Chest X-ray | ✓ | | LK |
| ECG | ✓ | | LK |
| Special tests | | Upper GI | LK |
| NPO as ordered | ✓ | | LK |
| Skin preparation | LK | ✓ 11/21 | 6 a.m. |
| Vital signs | LK | ✓ 130/84-76-18 | T-98 |
| Dentures removed | | ✓ none | LK |
| Prostheses removed | | ✓ none | LK |
| Jewelry removed | | ✓ ring taped | LK |
| Makeup, nail polish removed | ✓ | | LK |
| Voided | ✓ LK | | LK JD |
| Preanesthetic medication ordered | ✓ | | LK JD |

Drugs and dosages _Nembutal 50 mg I.M.,_
_Demerol 50 mg I.M., Atropine 0.4 mg I.M._
Time medicated _8:15 a.m._

By whom _Joyce Dobler, GN_

Unit nurse _Linda Kratz, R.N._

Operating room nurse _____

3. Nursing responsibilities
   a. Tell the patient why preoperative procedures are necessary
   b. Execute and document orders as indicated
   c. Obtain results of diagnostic tests, and alert the surgeon to abnormalities
   d. Note the date and time of I.V. cannulation and administration of I.V. fluids or medications
   e. Address the patient's and family members' questions and concerns

## E. Informed consent
1. General information
   a. Informed consent implies that the patient has been provided basic information about the surgery in language that he can understand
   b. Obtaining the patient's consent for elective or urgent surgery is a legal requirement that must be met before the patient undergoes the procedure but can be waived in emergencies, when the patient is in danger of losing life or limb
   c. The surgeon is responsible for obtaining informed consent, but most hospitals require the nurse to verify that informed consent has been given before transporting the patient to the operating room
   d. Informed consent is most commonly documented on a hospital form but can also be documented in the progress notes by the surgeon
   e. In most institutions, the nurse witnesses the patient's signature on the informed consent document
2. Nursing responsibilities
   a. Witness the patient's signature on the consent form only after the surgeon has discussed the procedure with the patient
   b. Inform the surgeon of anything that the patient does not understand
   c. Ensure that consent forms are accurately completed, witnessed, dated, and signed by the responsible parties
   d. Do not administer a preoperative sedative unless the patient's signature has been obtained; the validity of informed consent can be challenged if the patient signs the form after being sedated
   e. Alert the surgeon if the patient has been sedated before consent is obtained, and carefully document events that follow because of the increased possibility of litigation

## F. Preanesthesia evaluation
1. General information
   a. Every patient scheduled for anesthesia is seen preoperatively by a member of the anesthesia team (preferably the person who will administer the anesthetic), except when impractical, such as in an emergency
   b. A properly conducted preanesthesia visit enables the examiner to establish rapport, calm the patient (anxiety can cause catecholamine production, leading to hypertension and arrhythmias), and provide emotional support while assessing his emotional and physical status

    c. The preanesthesia evaluation includes discussion of alternative anesthetic techniques when feasible, a review of the risks and benefits of these techniques, instructions on the importance of compliance with NPO and other preoperative orders, a review of anticipated perioperative events, and verification that the patient understands the anesthesia plans

    d. Patients with special religious practices or beliefs, such as Jehovah's Witnesses, must be identified and counselled about options if they refuse blood transfusions

    e. The American Society of Anesthesiologists (ASA) has developed a system of classifying the patient's physical status preoperatively: the higher the assigned number, the higher the patient's risk under anesthesia; an "E" beside the status designation denotes emergency surgery

    f. Knowledge of the ASA classification helps the nurse anticipate and prepare for perioperative complications that may arise (see *Physical status classification for anesthesia*)

2. Patient history

    a. Knowledge of the patient's current and previous illnesses and surgery, anesthetic history, physical condition, and current drug use is essential to choosing the appropriate anesthetic

    b. The *history of current illness* examines factors responsible for and leading to the need for surgery

    c. Nausea, vomiting, and fever may dehydrate and weaken the patient

    d. Trauma patients must be assessed for the nature of the injury requiring intervention and other occult injuries, duration of any loss of consciousness, injury to the cervical spine, blood loss, chest or myocardial injury, burns, and musculoskeletal injury

    e. Obstetric patients must be assessed for complications of pregnancy; those with chronic or acute illness should be stabilized before surgery

    f. The *history of previous illness or surgery* includes the nature and type of prior illness or surgery that may affect the choice of anesthetic, such as cancer surgery followed by chemotherapy with bleomycin (Blenoxane) and adriamycin (Doxorubicin); bleomycin can cause oxygen toxicity and adriamycin is cardiotoxic

    g. The *anesthetic history* examines the patient's expectations, specific medical conditions, and previous experience with anesthesia

    h. The *review of systems* examines major body systems for current and previous illnesses or injuries

    i. Central nervous system: a history of seizures can influence the choice of inhalation agents; limitations from a previous stroke should be known before surgery, because weakness in an extremity may affect the patient's ability to move from stretcher to bed and influence the nurse's evaluation of recovery from regional anesthesia

---

## PHYSICAL STATUS CLASSIFICATION FOR ANESTHESIA

The following chart presents the American Society of Anesthesiologists' physical status descriptions for patients undergoing anesthesia.

| STATUS | DESCRIPTION |
|--------|-------------|
| P1 | A normal, healthy patient |
| P2 | A patient with mild systemic disease (such as heart disease that only slightly limits physical activity, essential hypertension, diabetes mellitus, anemia, extremes of age, morbid obesity, chronic bronchitis) |
| P3 | A patient with severe systemic disease (such as heart disease that limits activity, poorly controlled essential hypertension, diabetes mellitus with vascular complications, chronic pulmonary disease that limits activity, angina pectoris, history of myocardial infarction) |
| P4 | A patient with severe systemic disease that is a constant threat to life (such as congestive heart failure, persistent angina pectoris, advanced pulmonary, renal, or hepatic dysfunction) |
| P5 | A moribund patient who is not expected to survive without the operation (such as uncontrolled hemorrhage as from a ruptured abdominal aneurysm, cerebral trauma, pulmonary embolus) |
| P6 | A declared brain-dead patient whose organs are being removed for donation |

Adapted with permission from The American Society of Anesthesiologists, *Relative Value Guide 1990.*

---

    j.  Cardiovascular system: elective surgery should not be performed within 6 months of a myocardial infarction; hypertension or angina should be well controlled; patients with valvular disorders should be in optimal condition and may need antibiotic prophylaxis

    k.  Respiratory system: asthma can be aggravated by stress associated with hospitalization and surgery; smokers are at increased risk for postoperative pulmonary complications

    l.  Endocrine system: diabetes should be managed by an internist perioperatively; hyperthyroidism can be exacerbated by the stress of surgery; women of childbearing age should not undergo surgery until pregnancy is ruled out

    m.  Musculoskeletal system: arthritis may impair the mobility of the cervical spine and result in difficult intubation; myalgias and arthralgias may influence positioning during surgery

    n.  Hepatic and gastrointestinal systems: a history of hepatitis should be made known to minimize risk to the surgical team; hepatitis may influence the choice of inhalation agent; alcohol abuse can increase anesthetic requirements; gastroesophageal reflux or hiatal hernia increases the risk of aspiration

    o.  *Current drug use* includes prescription and nonprescription medications

    p.  The patient must reveal all current drug use, and allergies to medications must be noted on the patient's record to avoid anaphylactic reactions

    q.  Illegal drugs, especially such stimulants as cocaine, can interact with anesthetics and other drugs, causing cardiac arrest

    r.  Previously prescribed drugs, especially cardiotonic and antihypertensive agents, are usually continued throughout the perioperative period to maintain the patient's serum drug level

    s.  Use of nonprescription medications, such as ibuprofen (Advil), that can affect clotting and cough or cold preparations that can affect wakefulness should be documented

3.  Physical examination

    a.  The physical examination is conducted to evaluate the patient's overall condition, to note any conditions that may affect the anesthesia plan, and to obtain information that the patient has forgotten or neglected to reveal

    b.  The patient's general appearance is noted, as well as affects and mannerisms that may indicate anxiety

    c.  Evaluation of the airway includes assessment of the range of motion and position and shape of surrounding structures

    d.  Range of motion of the temporomandibular joint is evaluated to assess potential difficulties in endotracheal intubation; the mouth should open at least 3 fingerbreadths to permit use of laryngoscope and endotracheal tubes

    e.  Range of motion of the cervical spine is evaluated; the patient should be able to touch chin to chest and extend head on spine to facilitate endotracheal intubation

    f.  Position of mandible and shape of neck are noted; a receding mandible or short, thick neck may indicate difficult intubation

    g.  Excessive facial hair is noted; men with beards are hard to ventilate by mask because the seal is difficult to maintain and leaks develop around the edges of the mask

    h.  Arms and legs are evaluated for swelling, pain, discoloration, and condition of veins

    i.  Collateral circulation is evaluated if invasive arterial monitoring from any extremity is planned

    j.  Pain and tenderness must be documented preoperatively to help position the patient during surgery and direct the nurse's attention to special patient needs during ambulation or transferral from bed to stretcher

    k.  Presence of prostheses, contact lenses, or wigs is noted; capped, crowned, false, or loose teeth must be identified because they are more easily dislodged by airways or laryngoscope than natural teeth; the possibility of damage from intubation or airways should be mentioned to the patient

    l.  For regional anesthesia, the puncture site is inspected for access, inflammation, or conditions that might contraindicate the technique, and the patient's ability to assume the necessary position for spinal anesthesia is evaluated

4. Diagnostic studies
   a. The diagnostic studies required for a preoperative patient vary among institutions, may be influenced by the patient's insurance company, and should be ordered according to the patient's condition and planned surgery
   b. Typical preoperative tests include an ECG, blood studies, chest X-ray, and pulmonary function studies
   c. Hematology values, including white blood cell and platelet counts, are necessary because they may affect plans for regional anesthesia
   d. A hematocrit value of 30% or a hemoglobin level of 10 g/dl is generally considered the minimum acceptable for elective surgery
   e. Chemistry profiles include electrolyte values, liver enzymes, serum glucose, and renal function studies
   f. Pulmonary function testing is usually ordered for a patient with lung disease to establish a baseline for perioperative management

## Points to Remember

Failure to identify a patient can lead to inappropriate surgical procedures with potentially disastrous consequences.

A patient is shaved as close to the time of surgery as possible to avoid microbial colonization in nicked areas at the proposed surgical site.

The preoperative nursing assessment provides valuable baseline information that cannot be obtained from a sedated or unconscious patient.

Informed consent is required for all elective or urgent procedures, and the patient must sign a consent form before preoperative sedation.

A thorough preanesthesia evaluation enhances the probability of safe anesthetic administration and may reduce patient anxiety.

Certain medical and surgical conditions — as well as the patient's previous experience with anesthesia — influence the choice of anesthetic.

Medications routinely prescribed before surgery, especially cardiotonic and antihypertensive agents, should be continued throughout the perioperative period.

## Glossary

**Accessory muscles** — chest wall muscles not normally needed for respiration; use of these muscles during inspiration or forced expiration indicates breathing difficulty

**Cathartics** — medications or solutions used to facilitate evacuation of intestinal contents

**Endotracheal intubation** — passage of a tube through the mouth or nose into the trachea to facilitate breathing

**Gastroesophageal reflux** — return of solids or gastric secretions into the esophagus from the stomach, usually caused by hiatal hernia; places the patient at risk for aspiration during surgery

**Peritoneal cavity** — area containing all abdominal organs except the kidneys and bordered by the parietal peritoneum, the serous membrane that lines the abdominal and pelvic walls and the undersurface of the diaphragm

# Preoperative Medication

## Learning Objectives

After studying this section, the reader should be able to:

- State the purpose of preoperative medication.

- Name the classes of medication commonly prescribed before anesthesia.

- Discuss nursing responsibilities relevant to each class of medication.

- Identify the patient at risk for aspiration and describe aspiration prophylaxis.

## V. Preoperative Medication

### A. Introduction

1. The purpose of preoperative medication is to prepare the patient for anesthesia and surgery (see *Selected preoperative medications,* page 43)
2. Two or three preoperative medications are usually administered concomitantly to:
   a. Relieve anxiety
   b. Facilitate induction of anesthesia
   c. Reduce secretions in the oropharynx
   d. Inhibit stimulation of the vagus nerve
   e. Reduce the possibility of aspiration of gastric contents or secretions
   f. Minimize damage to the lungs in the event of aspiration
3. Classes of preoperative medication include:
   a. Narcotics
   b. Agonist-antagonists
   c. Barbiturates
   d. Antianxiety agents
   e. Anticholinergic agents
   f. Antacids and other agents
4. The class of medication prescribed and the dose administered are determined by the patient's:
   a. Age and weight
   b. Physical condition
   c. Anxiety level
   d. Tolerance of depressant drugs
   e. Previous experience with the drug
   f. Type of surgery
5. Preoperative medications are administered by several routes, including:
   a. Oral, with a sip of water
   b. Intramuscular injection
   c. Intravenous injection
   d. Subcutaneous injection
   e. Nasal instillation
6. Prescription medications routinely taken by the patient should be continued throughout the perioperative period to maintain the patient's serum drug level
7. Medication to prevent or reduce damage from aspiration of gastric contents is typically prescribed for outpatients, trauma patients, patients with hiatal hernia, and obstetric patients
8. Preoperative medications are usually given 60 to 90 minutes before surgery
   a. The anesthetist may specify the time of administration
   b. The medication may be ordered *on call* (a surgical team member calls the nurse when the medication should be administered)

9. No preoperative medications should be given until all consent forms have been signed and are in order
   a. A patient is not considered competent to sign a consent form after receiving preoperative medication
   b. Family members cannot sign for a patient unless they are legal guardians
10. General nursing responsibilities include:
   a. Assessing the patient's anxiety level the night before surgery and offering sedatives, if ordered
   b. Ensuring that the consent form has been signed and that all necessary information appears on the chart before administering preoperative medication
   c. Having the patient empty his bladder before administering preoperative medication and instructing the medicated patient to stay in bed and not get up without assistance
   d. Putting the bed in the lowest position, raising side rails, and placing the call button within reach to promote patient safety and reduce incidence of falls
   e. Obtaining baseline vital signs and determining level of consciousness before administering preoperative medication, and monitoring and documenting the medication's effect 10 to 20 minutes after intramuscular injection or 30 to 45 minutes after oral administration
   f. Assisting with transfer of the patient from hospital bed to stretcher after rechecking the patient's identification and chart to ensure that all information is documented

B. **Narcotics**
   1. General information
      a. Prescribed preoperatively, usually by intramuscular injection, to relieve the pain of current medical conditions and to provide analgesia for painful procedures, such as insertion of I.V. lines
      b. Are most effective when given before painful procedures or before pain becomes intense
      c. Help minimize the patient's perception of pain
      d. Facilitate the induction of anesthesia by blunting the stress response, causing some patients to become euphoric
      e. Decrease the amount of anesthetic required and depress respirations in a dose-dependent manner
      f. Can be reversed by the narcotic antagonist naloxone (Narcan) or a narcotic agonist-antagonist
   2. Mechanism of action
      a. Produce analgesia by stimulating opioid receptors in the brain and spinal cord
      b. Alter perception and emotional response to pain
   3. Uses
      a. Perioperative analgesia
      b. Facilitation of anesthesia induction (blunts the sympathetic response)

4. Contraindications
   a. Allergy to drug
   b. Somnolence or unresponsiveness
   c. Respiratory depression
5. Complications
   a. Respiratory depression, including hypoxia, hypercapnia, and possibly death
   b. Nausea and vomiting
   c. Itching caused by histamine release
   d. Orthostatic hypotension
   e. Biliary colic (may be precipitated or aggravated by meperidine)
6. Examples
   a. Morphine
   b. Meperidine (Demerol)
   c. Hydromorphone (Dilaudid)
7. Nursing responsibilities
   a. Check the availability of a narcotic antagonist, such as naloxone, before administering a narcotic
   b. Inform the patient that constipation is a common postoperative side effect of narcotic administration, and ask the physician to order stool softeners, if necessary

C. **Agonist-antagonists**
   1. General information
      a. Stimulate (agonist) and inhibit (antagonist) opioid receptors
      b. Provide some sedative and antianxiety effects and are administered by intramuscular injection
      c. Can precipitate withdrawal symptoms (increased sensory perceptions, yawning, sweating, facial flushing, muscle spasms) and worsen pain in a patient addicted to narcotics or dependent on them for pain control
   2. Mechanism of action
      a. May bind to opioid receptors, competing for the opiate receptors in the brain that alter pain perception and response
      b. May depend on the amount of drug bound to the receptors and the presence of other opioid agonists
   3. Uses
      a. Analgesia
      b. Sedation
   4. Contraindications
      a. Sensitivity to drug
      b. Narcotic addiction
   5. Complications
      a. Dizziness and light-headedness
      b. Nausea and vomiting
      c. Acute withdrawal symptoms in narcotic-addicted patients

6. Examples
   a. Nalbuphine (Nubain)
   b. Butorphanol (Stadol)
   c. Pentazocine (Talwin)
7. Nursing responsibilities
   a. Check the availability of a narcotic antagonist (such as naloxone) before administering any narcotic agent in case respiratory depression develops
   b. Inform the patient that constipation may occur postoperatively with nalbuphine administration, and ask the physician to order stool softeners, if necessary
   c. Do not mix pentazocine and barbiturates in the same syringe because a precipitate will form
   d. Notify the physician if withdrawal symptoms occur, and institute safety precautions (raise side rails, have emergency equipment available, caution against ambulation or other activities requiring alertness)

D. **Barbiturates**
   1. General information
      a. Prescribed preoperatively to reduce anxiety and produce sedation; also given the night before surgery to promote sleep
      b. Cause minimal respiratory and circulatory depression in usual adult doses
      c. Now used infrequently for preoperative sedation because safer antianxiety agents, such as the benzodiazepines, are available
      d. Administered by mouth with a sip of water or by intramuscular injection
   2. Mechanism of action
      a. Depress the cerebral cortex, causing generalized central nervous system (CNS) depression
      b. Decrease presynaptic and postsynaptic membrane permeability
   3. Uses
      a. Preoperative sedation
      b. Relief of preoperative insomnia
   4. Contraindications
      a. Allergy to drug
      b. Porphyria
      c. Preexisting CNS depression
   5. Complications
      a. Paradoxical excitement, especially in the elderly patient
      b. Exacerbation of pain
      c. Allergic reactions caused by histamine release, especially in asthmatic patients
      d. Potentiation of other CNS depressants
   6. Examples
      a. Pentobarbital (Nembutal)
      b. Secobarbital (Seconal)

7. Nursing responsibilities
   a. Assess the patient's sleep state for drug effectiveness when barbiturates are used to relieve insomnia
   b. Institute safety precautions after medication is given (raise side rails, maintain bed rest, caution against performing activities that require alertness)
   c. Remember that an elderly patient may require a lower-than-recommended dose
   d. Assess elderly patients for agitation and disorientation, and calmly reorient patients to their surroundings
   e. Inject the medication into a large muscle mass to promote adequate absorption when giving barbiturates intramuscularly
   f. Do not mix secobarbital or pentobarbital with other medications in the same syringe because a precipitate will form
   g. Administer an intramuscular injection deeply; superficial injection may cause pain, sterile abscess, and tissue sloughing

**E. Antianxiety agents**
   1. General information
      a. Reduce a patient's fear and apprehension, resulting in smoother induction of anesthesia
      b. Have largely replaced barbiturates for preoperative sedation because they possess many of the same features but are safer (benzodiazepines)
      c. Administered by intramuscular injection or by mouth with a sip of water on the day of surgery
   2. Mechanism of action
      a. Interfere with CNS transmission at postsynaptic dopamine receptors
      b. Interfere with interneuronal transmission at the spinal cord and enhance the effects of gamma aminobutyric acid (benzodiazepines)
      c. Inhibit the medullary chemoreceptor trigger zone and act as antiemetics (phenothiazines and butyrophenones)
   3. Uses
      a. Preoperative sedation and anxiety relief
      b. Relief of nausea and vomiting during the perioperative period (phenothiazines, butyrophenones)
      c. Diminished recall of perioperative events (benzodiazepines)
   4. Contraindications
      a. Allergy to drug
      b. Pregnancy (fetal malformations can occur with benzodiazepine administration)
      c. Parkinson's disease
   5. Complications
      a. Exacerbation of Parkinson's disease or production of similar extrapyramidal symptoms (droperidol)
      b. Paradoxic reaction of agitation and anxiety rather than sedation

    c.  Respiratory depression when benzodiazepines are combined with such narcotics as midazolam (Versed), which has been associated with significant respiratory depression and death in patients, especially elderly or debilitated patients, who were not monitored closely

    d.  Hypotonia and jaundice in breast-feeding infants (benzodiazepines are excreted in breast milk)

    e.  Hypotension, especially orthostatic hypotension postoperatively

    f.  Inner storm, in which patient appears calm and detached but postoperatively reports agitation and anxiety (droperidol)

  6.  Examples

    a.  Benzodiazepines—diazepam (Valium), lorazepam (Ativan)

    b.  Butyrophenones—droperidol (Inapsine)

    c.  Phenothiazines—hydroxyzine (Vistaril), promethazine (Phenergan)

  7.  Nursing responsibilities

    a.  Keep in mind that antianxiety agents are not substitutes for compassion and communication

    b.  Try to determine and relieve the source of the patient's anxiety, using nonpharmacologic means when possible, such as talking and providing emotional support; do not administer an antianxiety agent until ordered and after other measures have failed to relieve the anxiety

    c.  Reorient the patient if amnesia occurs, to minimize patient upset and distress

**F.  Anticholinergic agents**

  1.  General information

    a.  Administered preoperatively by intramuscular injection to decrease secretions in the oropharynx and reduce incidence of vagal-induced bradycardia during laryngoscopy and surgery

    b.  Depress the parasympathetic nervous system, resulting in increased heart rate, and elevate body temperature

    c.  Reduces postoperative nausea and vomiting in some patients (scopolamine)

    d.  Do not cross the blood-brain barrier or placenta (glycopyrrolate)

    e.  Do not increase intraocular pressure when given in recommended doses and are usually acceptable for the patient with glaucoma

  2.  Mechanism of action

    a.  Block the action of acetylcholine within the parasympathetic nervous system

    b.  Block the vagus nerve

    c.  Stimulate the cerebral cortex (except glycopyrrolate)

  3.  Uses

    a.  Decrease incidence of vagal-induced bradycardia during surgery and laryngoscopy

    b.  Reduce secretions

  4.  Contraindications

    a.  Sensitivity to drug

      b. Narrow angle glaucoma
      c. Obstructive uropathy
      d. Myasthenia gravis
      e. Obstructive GI tract disease

  5. Complications
      a. Excitement and agitation (atropine and scopolamine cross the blood-brain barrier), which are usually relieved by physostigmine (Antilirium)
      b. Heat retention and elevated body temperature
      c. Urine retention
      d. Blurred vision

  6. Examples
      a. Scopolamine (Buscospan)
      b. Atropine
      c. Glycopyrrolate (Robinul)

  7. Nursing responsibilities
      a. Be aware that black patients may require higher doses because of increased secretions
      b. Tell the patient that his mouth may become dry, and instruct him not to chew gum or suck on hard candy because these activities may stimulate gastric acid secretion
      c. Remember that heart rate normally increases after injection; this response is not significant unless the rate is excessively higher than the preinjection rate
      d. Reassure the patient and notify the physician if excitement or agitation occurs
      e. Assess urine retention after drug administration, and alert the physician if routine nursing measures (such as ensuring privacy and running water) do not induce urination
      f. Tell the patient that his vision may blur, and encourage him to avoid reading or other activities that require focusing the eyes

## G. Antacids and other agents
  1. General information
      a. Antacids and other agents are used in aspiration prophylaxis, an important precaution because aspiration of only 25 ml of gastric secretions with a pH of 2.5 or less during anesthesia can produce a fatal pneumonia
      b. Those at risk for aspiration include pregnant patients, trauma patients, outpatients, patients with hiatal hernia or symptoms of reflux, and patients who have recently eaten
      c. Preoperative aspiration prophylaxis typically consists of administering a *GI stimulant,* such as metoclopramide, 1 hour before surgery to promote stomach emptying; an *antacid* just before surgery to immediately raise the pH of the stomach; and a *histamine ($H_2$) receptor antagonist* to maintain a higher pH

## SELECTED PREOPERATIVE MEDICATIONS

Many combinations of drugs are used preoperatively, but the most common one is a narcotic combined with an antianxiety agent and anticholinergic agent. The following are commonly administered preoperative medications, dosages, and their actions. Before administration, the nurse should explain the drug effects to the patient, provide privacy by closing the curtains, and ensure safety by pulling up the bed side rails.

| DRUG | DOSAGE | ACTION |
| --- | --- | --- |
| **Narcotic agonists** | | |
| meperidine (Demerol) | 50 to 100 mg I.M. or S.C. 30 to 90 minutes before surgery | Alters perception and emotional response to pain |
| morphine | 8 to 12 mg I.M. 30 to 90 minutes before surgery | Alters perception and emotional response to pain |
| **Barbiturates** | | |
| pentobarbital (Nembutal) | 150 to 200 mg I.M. 40 to 60 minutes before surgery | Sedates |
| secobarbital (Seconal) | 200 to 300 mg P.O. 1 to 2 hours before surgery | Sedates |
| **Anticholinergics** | | |
| atropine | 0.4 to 0.6 mg I.M. 45 to 60 minutes before surgery | Reduces secretions, vomiting, and laryngospasm |
| scopolamine (Buscospan) | 0.4 to 0.6 mg S.C. 45 to 60 minutes before surgery | Reduces secretions, vomiting, and laryngospasm |
| **Antianxiety agents** | | |
| diazepam (Valium) | 5 to 10 mg I.V. immediately before surgery | Sedates |
| hydroxyzine (Vistaril) | 25 to 100 mg I.M. 30 to 60 minutes before surgery | Reduces anxiety |

2. Mechanism of action
   a. Buffer and neutralize gastric hydrochloric acid (antacids) but may contain particulates that damage the lungs if aspirated (magnesium and aluminum hydroxide)
   b. Competitively inhibit the action of histamine at $H_2$ receptors to reduce gastric acid secretion ($H_2$ receptor antagonists)
   c. Promote motility and emptying of the GI tract by increasing the tone and amplitude of gastric contractions (GI stimulants)
3. Uses
   a. Reduce the potential for aspiration during anesthesia
   b. Control nausea and vomiting

4.  Contraindications
    a.  Sensitivity to any of the agents
    b.  Mechanical obstruction or perforation of the GI tract
    c.  Seizure disorder (metoclopramide)
5.  Complications
    a.  Extrapyramidal reactions (metoclopramide)
    b.  Nausea and vomiting (antacids)
6.  Examples
    a.  Antacid — sodium citrate and citric acid solution (Bicitra), magnesium and aluminum hydroxide (Maalox)
    b.  $H_2$ antagonist — cimetidine (Tagamet), ranitidine (Zantac)
    c.  GI stimulant — metoclopramide (Reglan)
7.  Nursing responsibilities
    a.  Inform the patient of the reasons for aspiration prophylaxis, and stress the importance of complying with nothing-by-mouth orders
    b.  Advise the patient to call for assistance before getting out of bed because metoclopramide can cause drowsiness
    c.  Administer aspiration prophylaxis at the precise times ordered to achieve maximum effect

## Points to Remember

Preoperative medication should not be administered until the patient has signed all consent forms.

Agonist-antagonists can precipitate withdrawal symptoms in patients dependent on narcotics.

When feasible, antianxiety agents should not be administered until the source of the patient's anxiety has been sought and nonpharmacologic measures have failed to relieve it.

## Glossary

**Anticholinergic drugs** — pharmacologic agents that act against the parasympathetic system to inhibit secretions and block the reflex slowing of the heart rate caused by vagal stimulation

**Aspiration** — regurgitation of gastric secretions into the lungs, causing damage on contact and possible airway obstruction

**Porphyria** — congenital metabolic disease associated with abdominal pain, psychiatric manifestations, and reddish urine; exacerbated by barbiturates

**Vagus nerve** — tenth cranial nerve, responsible for inhibiting increases in heart rate but can cause bradycardia when stimulated

# Types of Anesthesia

## Learning Objectives

After studying this section, the reader should be able to:

- Define anesthesia.

- Identify indications for local, regional, and general anesthesia.

- Discuss methods of inducing regional anesthesia.

- Describe nursing responsibilities relevant to each type of anesthesia.

## VI. Types of Anesthesia

### A. Introduction

1. *Anesthesia* ("without sensation") is classified according to the site and degree of sensory loss
2. The three major types of anesthesia are local, regional, and general
3. Drugs are used to produce anesthesia, which may or may not be accompanied by loss of consciousness
4. Balanced anesthesia requires a combination of drugs to produce a loss of sensation while maximizing the drugs' benefits and minimizing their side effects

### B. Local anesthesia

1. General information
   a. Produces loss of sensation at a specific site after injection of local anesthetics near certain nerves or infiltration of the agents into a specific area, thus blocking sensory nerve branches
   b. Can also be induced by topical anesthetic that paralyzes nerve endings
   c. Does not affect mental activity (in usual adult doses), and the patient remains aware of conversations
   d. Is used for cataract surgery; pacemaker implantation; indwelling central catheter insertion; and some neurologic, otolaryngologic, and gynecologic procedures, including nasal surgery, craniotomy, and dilatation and curettage
   e. Usually does not necessitate anesthesia personnel in attendance during surgery
2. Conscious sedation
   a. Is used when surgery is performed under local anesthesia
   b. Reduces anxiety and pain; patient usually remains responsive
   c. Should be administered only by trained personnel who are familiar with the drugs used and who are prepared to deal with such adverse reactions as seizures, apnea, and cardiac arrest
3. Nursing responsibilities
   a. Restrain conversation because patients usually remain aware of their surroundings
   b. Monitor the patient's level of consciousness and vital signs
   c. Have at hand suction, oxygen, airway management equipment (manual resuscitation bag, laryngoscope, endotracheal tube, oral and nasal airways), and resuscitative drugs should an adverse reaction occur
   d. Ensure that the patient takes nothing by mouth (apnea and seizures are possible consequences of local anesthetics, and fatal aspiration can occur if the patient has eaten)

## C. Regional anesthesia
1. General information
   a. Produces loss of sensation in a specific area or region of the body; also referred to as a *block*
   b. Is accomplished by injecting local anesthetics into specific nerves to block nerve impulses; the size and location of the anesthetized area depend on the application site and on the amount, concentration, and penetrating ability of the anesthetic agent
   c. Allows patients to remain awake and in control of their airways
   d. Is safe; ordinarily, physiologic nerve function is completely restored, yet some patients fear permanent paralysis and backaches from spinal and epidural anesthesia
   e. Has no systemic effects and is a rational choice for surgery on a specific body part, such as an extremity, and during childbirth when the anesthetic's effect on the fetus and neonate must be considered
   f. Is not commonly used for children because they are seldom able to cooperate with injection of the anesthetic agents
2. Spinal anesthesia (subarachnoid block)
   a. Induces loss of sensation after injection of a local anesthetic into the lumbar region of the spine, blocking transmissions from sensory, motor, and autonomic nerve fibers
   b. May cause headache, hypotension, bradycardia, and cardiovascular collapse
   c. Is administered in a single dose to patient sitting or lying on his side, with head tucked and knees flexed to open the interlaminar spaces
   d. Mixes anesthetic agent with cerebrospinal fluid (CSF) to bathe the nerves, rapidly blocking conduction and causing prompt onset of anesthesia
   e. Is affected by the amount and type of local anesthetic injected and the patient's position during and after injection
   f. Blocks nerves also used to control vasomotor tone, dilating the vasculature in the affected area and decreasing blood pressure (hypotension can be blunted by an I.V. bolus of 500 to 1,000 ml of fluid administered before the block)
   g. Numbs areas that would touch a saddle (known as a *saddle block*) when administered in small amounts to a sitting patient; induces anesthesia to the level of the nipples when administered in larger amounts to a supine patient (used for cesarean section)
   h. May cause spinal headache because the dura (the sac that encloses the spinal cord) is punctured to administer the anesthetic and CSF may leak out, reducing the volume of CSF available in the skull to cushion the brain; when the patient stands, the gravitational pull on the brain causes a positional headache that resolves when the patient lies down
   i. Is used for childbirth, cesarean section, and surgery involving the legs, abdomen (appendectomy or hernia repair), or perineum

    j.  Is contraindicated in uncooperative or disruptive patients and those with hypovolemia, poorly controlled heart disease, clotting abnormalities or use of anticoagulant drugs, infection or anomaly at the injection site, increased intracranial pressure, or systemic sepsis

    k.  Can result in *high spinal anesthesia* (when the local anesthetic spreads farther along the spinal cord than planned and impairs muscles associated with respiration) or *total spinal anesthesia* (when the local anesthetic spreads throughout the spinal cord, causing apnea and unconsciousness)

3.  Epidural anesthesia

    a.  Induces loss of sensation after injection of a local anesthetic into the epidural space, diffusing the anesthetic into the subarachnoid space and blocking the spinal nerve roots

    b.  Is less reliable than spinal anesthesia because diffusion rates vary and can produce patchy or inadequate anesthesia

    c.  Can be performed at any site along the spinal cord — caudal, lumbar (most common), thoracic, or cervical — and is administered to a patient sitting or lying with his back curved

    d.  Is determined by the concentration and volume of the local anesthetic and the location of the injection along the spinal cord

    e.  Can be administered as a single injection but usually involves placement of a catheter into the epidural space for repeated doses or continuous infusion

    f.  Takes longer to induce than spinal anesthesia because it involves placing a catheter and injecting a test dose of local anesthetic before the recommended dose is given

    g.  Allows anesthetics to be added as necessary through the catheter, a benefit when surgery runs longer than anticipated (the catheter is not left in place more than 72 hours because of the risk of infection)

    h.  Has a slower onset of action than spinal anesthesia, so blood pressure usually remains stable

    i.  Does not cause positional headache unless the dura is inadvertently punctured

    j.  Is used for childbirth, cesarean section, surgery on the legs or abdomen, skin grafts on the legs, postoperative pain relief, and relief of painful chronic conditions, such as backache

    k.  Is contraindicated in cases similar to those for spinal anesthesia

    l.  Narcotics and steroids can be injected into the epidural space to relieve chronic or perioperative pain

4.  Intravenous regional anesthesia (Bier block)

    a.  Induces loss of sensation after injection of a local anesthetic into the veins of an extremity, which is exsanguinated by wrapping it with an elastic bandage and inflating a tourniquet to occlude venous flow and prevent the anesthetic from entering the systemic circulation

b. Produces loss of sensation in about 10 minutes and lasts for 1 to 2 hours
c. Is used for soft tissue procedures below the elbow or knee, such as ganglionectomy, carpal tunnel repair, and excision of neuromas
d. Is contraindicated when patient has an allergy to the local anesthetic
e. Can cause seizures from rapid release of the tourniquet, allowing a large volume of local anesthetic to surge into the systemic circulation

5. Nerve block
   a. Induces loss of sensation after injection of a local anesthetic solution at or near specific nerves that conduct impulses to the brain
   b. May be used alone or with other anesthetic techniques to control perioperative pain and can be induced continuously with an indwelling catheter
   c. Can block almost any nerve when performed by a skilled practitioner; in less experienced hands, may provide inadequate anesthesia for surgery
   d. Is commonly used in the brachial plexus, cervical plexus, and intercostal nerves
   e. Can also be used in the radial, ulnar, and digital nerves; known as *peripheral nerve block*
   f. Is used for surgery on the extremities and relief of chronic pain
   g. Is contraindicated in cases of patient inability to cooperate with placement of the block and surgical procedures lasting more than 1 to 2 hours
   h. Can cause seizures and cardiovascular collapse (if local anesthetics are inadvertently injected into the circulation), pneumothorax (from intercostal block of nerves in the chest), hematomas at the injection site, and neuropathy

6. Nursing responsibilities
   a. Clarify inaccurate perceptions (many patients fear paralysis after regional anesthesia), but tell the patient that complications are possible with any anesthesia
   b. Notify the anesthesia team of the patient's apprehensions, and comfort the patient during the procedure to alleviate anxiety
   c. Reassure the patient that he will remain awake for the surgery but will not observe the operation
   d. Explain that sedatives diminish recall of perioperative events
   e. Verify that the patient has taken nothing by mouth — general anesthesia may be needed if the regional block is inadequate or the patient becomes restless and uncooperative
   f. Obtain the necessary equipment, including antiseptic solution, supply kit (some institutions use disposable equipment trays), and appropriate local anesthetics; ensure that suction, oxygen, and airway management equipment are available should complications occur
   g. Attach blood pressure cuff and electrocardiogram leads, if necessary, and position the patient to facilitate administration of the anesthetic

h. Administer I.V. fluids as ordered—a bolus of 500 to 1,000 ml is commonly infused before spinal anesthesia to counteract hypotension seen after induction

i. Check tourniquets before use during I.V. regional anesthesia because sudden deflation of a tourniquet can cause a seizure

j. Assist the anesthesia team if a seizure occurs by securing the patient's position on the table, obtaining necessary drugs or supplies, and maintaining the airway to prevent hypoxic injury

k. Label epidural catheters used for postoperative and labor pain relief and never inject anything into them, which could destroy the spinal cord or nerves

l. Notify the anesthesia team if the patient receives anticoagulant therapy so that the catheter can be removed to prevent bleeding into the epidural space

m. Assist the anesthesia team with intubation if total spinal anesthesia occurs; the patient must be manually or mechanically ventilated with oxygen until able to breathe independently

n. Unless ordered otherwise, instruct the patient recovering from spinal anesthesia to lie flat for 12 to 24 hours after surgery; the patient can have a pillow under his head but cannot sit up to eat or drink (offer liquids through a straw) or get up to use the bathroom

o. Disconnect electrical beds to prevent inadvertent raising of the head

p. Notify the anesthesia team and surgeon if spinal headache develops

q. Administer analgesics as ordered to minimize patient discomfort while awaiting the anesthesia team's evaluation

r. Evaluate the patient for urine retention after spinal anesthesia, and palpate the abdomen to reduce patient discomfort and risk of urinary tract infection; notify the physician if bladder distention occurs or if patient cannot void

## D. General anesthesia

1. General information

   a. Is a state of altered physiology characterized by amnesia, analgesia, and muscle relaxation that is usually produced by a combination of intravenous and inhaled drugs

   b. Reduces the catecholamine-induced stress response to surgical pain and must be deep enough to prevent patient movement but not so deep that cardiovascular collapse results

   c. Renders the patient unconscious, insensible to pain, and without muscle tone and reflexes

   d. Has four stages: analgesia, excitement, surgical anesthesia, and medullary paralysis (see *Stages of general anesthesia,* page 52)

## STAGES OF GENERAL ANESTHESIA

General anesthesia can progress through the four stages described below. Originally developed to describe ether anesthesia, the stages vary, depending on the anesthetic used, induction speed, and the anesthetist's skill.

| STAGE | DESCRIPTION | CHARACTERISTICS |
|---|---|---|
| I. Analgesia | • Begins with onset of anesthesia<br>• Ends with loss of consciousness | • Loss of sense of smell and pain perception<br>• Exaggerated hearing<br>• Possible hallucinations and dreams<br>• Slurred speech<br>• Numbness that spreads over the body |
| II. Excitement | • Begins with loss of consciousness<br>• Ends with loss of eyelid reflexes | • Irregular respirations<br>• Increased autonomic activity<br>• Exaggerated reflexes |
| III. Surgical anesthesia | • Begins with loss of eyelid reflexes<br>• Ends with respiratory paralysis | • Diminished reflexes<br>• Relaxed muscle tone<br>• Normalization of respirations<br>• Constricted pupils and sluggish reaction to light<br>• Decreased body temperature |
| IV. Medullary paralysis | • Begins with respiratory paralysis<br>• Ends with apnea and death | • Loss of respirations<br>• Collapse of circulatory system<br>• Mechanical ventilation required |

e. Consists of three phases: *induction* (begins with administration of the anesthetic agent and continues until the patient is unconscious and ready for skin preparation, incision, or surgical manipulation; intubation is performed if necessary; corresponds to the stages of analgesia and excitement), *maintenance* (begins with loss of consciousness and involves administration of inhaled agents or titrated doses of I.V. drugs until surgery nears completion), and *emergence* (begins with termination of the anesthetic administration and varies in duration, usually ending when the patient responds to commands and is ready to leave the operating room; extubation is performed)

f. Requires monitoring of the patient's blood pressure and heart rate and rhythm, and additional monitoring is recommended to assess the patient's respiratory and neurologic status

    g. Is used for operations lasting longer than 1 to 2 hours; operations requiring prone, lateral, or unique positions in which access to the patient's airway is limited; most pediatric cases; and emergency surgery, such as obstetric and trauma cases

    h. Is recommended for patients who are uncooperative because of pain, dementia, intoxication, or disorientation

    i. Is contraindicated in patients who have ingested food or fluids within 6 hours of surgery

    j. Is not advised for patients with esophageal reflux, abnormal blood tests, history of heart disease or myocardial infarction within the past 6 months, history of lung disease, family history of malignant hyperthermia, or poorly controlled conditions (such as diabetes, hypertension, or kidney failure)

    k. Can cause aspiration of stomach contents into the lungs; damage to teeth, lips, or vocal cords from intubation or use of artificial airways; damage to eyes from drying or pressure from surgeon or instruments resting on them; damage to peripheral nerves from positioning, retractors, or surgical team leaning on patient; malignant hyperthermia; arrhythmias; hypoxia; and cardiovascular collapse

2. Nursing responsibilities: Induction

    a. Reassure the patient that using multiple anesthetics is routine and typically does not adversely affect the body

    b. Assist the anesthesia team and act as patient advocate to reduce patient anxiety, facilitate administration of anesthesia, and protect the patient from injury

    c. Maintain a quiet, professional environment to facilitate a smooth induction and calm the patient as needed (anxiety may peak during induction)

    d. Stand by to assist the anesthesia team until the airway is secure; surgery should not begin until this is accomplished

3. Nursing responsibilities: Maintenance

    a. Monitor the patient for hypothermia, a constant hazard during surgery and anesthesia because of exposed body cavities, excessively cool environment, use of cool inspired gases, and central nervous system effects of anesthesia

    b. Regulate room temperature to prevent overcooling; warm solutions, place warm blankets on the patient, and use a heating blanket on the surgical table to combat hypothermia

    c. Pause after each repositioning of the patient to allow the anesthesia team to evaluate patency of the airway or endotracheal tube; repositioning can dislodge these devices

    d. Prepare to assist the anesthesia team if vital signs change during the procedure

4. Nursing responsibilities: Emergence
   a. Provide a quiet environment, giving the patient gentle verbal and tactile reassurances (hearing is the first sense to return after anesthesia)
   b. Assist the anesthesia team as necessary with transfer to the recovery room by moving the patient slowly from the stretcher to minimize pain, motion sickness, and blood pressure swings
   c. Dress the patient in a clean gown if the original one is soiled, and preserve the patient's dignity as he regains consciousness
   d. Cover the patient with warm blankets to reduce heat loss

## Points to Remember

Conscious sedation should be administered only by those who are familiar with the drugs and who are prepared to resuscitate the patient if seizures, apnea, or cardiac arrest occurs.

Regional anesthesia is a safe alternative to general anesthesia for many patients, but unfounded fears of paralysis and observing the operation cause some patients to refuse this technique.

Spinal anesthesia involves a single injection of a local anesthetic beneath the dura into the CSF; it is generally easy to perform, prompt in onset, and reliable in producing loss of sensation.

Epidural anesthesia takes longer to achieve than spinal anesthesia and may produce spotty pain relief, but it produces more stable blood pressure levels. Intravenous regional anesthesia is induced by impeding the circulation within an extremity with a pneumatic tourniquet and injecting a local anesthetic into the isolated circulation.

Specific nerves can be blocked by skilled practitioners, but a nerve block may be inadequate for surgery and more useful for postoperative pain relief.

## Glossary

**Block** — any regional anesthetic technique

**Epidural space** — slender space above the spinal cord and outside the dura

**General anesthesia** — state of altered physiology characterized by amnesia, analgesia, and muscle relaxation

**Induction** — causing anesthesia, or loss of sensation, by administering anesthetic agents; encompasses the time from administration of the first agent to the onset of suitable anesthesia

**Infiltration** — diffusion of an injected drug through intracutaneous or subcutaneous tissue

**Intubation** — insertion of a tube through the mouth or nose into the trachea to maintain a patent airway

**Spinal headache** — headache resulting from CSF leakage through a puncture in the dura during spinal anesthetic administration; less CSF means less cushioning for the brain when the patient stands, causing pain from traction of sensitive structures

# Anesthetic Agents

**Learning Objectives**
After studying this section, the reader should be able to:

- Identify two classes of local anesthetic agents.

- Describe symptoms of local anesthetic toxicity.

- Name two I.V. drugs and three inhalation agents used in general anesthesia.

- Define carrier gases.

- Discuss nursing responsibilities relevant to each type of anesthetic agent.

# VII. Anesthetic Agents

A. **Amides and esters**
  1. General information
     a. Constitute the two types of local anesthetic agent: the ester cocaine was the first local anesthetic used in medicine (introduced in 1884 and used in spinal anesthesia in 1885); the amide lidocaine is injected intravenously to suppress cardiac arrhythmias
     b. Can be injected or applied topically to numb mucous membranes and afferent nerve endings
     c. Induce varying degrees of anesthesia, depending on the administration site, the agent's concentration, and the duration of contact with nerve tissues
     d. Diminish sensory reactions in specific order—loss of temperature sensation, blocking and eventual disappearance of pain sensation, dulling of tactile sense, blocking of motor impulses, and weakening of deep pressure sense; usually return in reverse order
  2. Mechanism of action
     a. Prevent generation and conduction of nerve impulses
     b. Decrease or prevent permeability of transient nerve cell membranes to sodium and potassium ions to block conduction
     c. Decrease electrical excitability of the myocardium (high concentrations can cause cardiac arrest or ventricular fibrillation)
     d. Interfere with the uptake of norepinephrine, producing sensitization to catecholamine seizures and possible cardiac arrest from overdosage
  3. Uses
     a. Local anesthesia
     b. Regional anesthesia
  4. Contraindications
     a. Allergy to agent
     b. Inflammation or infection in puncture region
  5. Complications
     a. Allergic reactions, though rare, include dermatitis, asthma, and fatal anaphylaxis
     b. Inadvertent I.V. injection can lead to toxicity, as evidenced by dizziness, tinnitus, somnolence, disorientation, hypotension, and bradycardia
     c. Severe toxicity results in ventricular arrhythmias, asystole, seizures, respiratory arrest, and unconsciousness
     d. Maternal or fetal death from local anesthetic toxicity can occur during labor
  6. Examples
     a. Amides—mepivacaine (Carbocaine), bupivacaine, (Marcaine), lidocaine (Xylocaine), and prilocaine (Citanest)
     b. Esters—procaine (Novocain), chloroprocaine (Nesacaine), tetracaine (Pontocaine), and cocaine

7. Nursing responsibilities
   a. Remember that only the smallest effective dose should be administered to minimize the risk of complications and adverse reactions
   b. Keep emergency drugs and resuscitation equipment at hand during administration of a local anesthetic in case of a toxic or allergic reaction
   c. Assess the anesthetic's effectiveness after administration by checking the patient's sensory functions
   d. Check the peripheral pulse, color, and temperature of the affected extremity, and compare that with the unaffected extremity when a local anesthetic is used for regional anesthesia
   e. Instruct a patient receiving a local anesthetic to protect the anesthetized area until sensation returns
   f. Check for return of the gag reflex before feeding a patient who has received a local anesthetic to the oropharyngeal mucosa
      (for additional nursing responsibilities, see *Comparing local anesthetic agents,* pages 59 and 60)

B. **Barbiturates**
   1. General information
      a. Are ultrashort-acting agents used in general anesthesia and usually followed by administration of inhaled or additional injected agents because of their short-lived effect
      b. Can be combined with inhaled nitrous oxide or oxygen to induce anesthesia for brief procedures
      c. Take effect in about 10 seconds (the time it takes blood to circulate from the arm to the brain) when administered by I.V. injection
      d. Are usually injected intravenously in adults to induce sedation or unconsciousness for 10 to 20 minutes and can be given rectally to children
   2. Mechanism of action
      a. Affect cerebral cortex and reticular activating system to cause sedation or unconsciousness, depending on the dose used
      b. Inhibit the firing rate of neurons within the ascending reticular activating system
   3. Uses
      a. Sedation
      b. Unconsciousness for anesthesia induction
   4. Contraindications
      a. Allergy to drug
      b. Porphyria
      c. Status asthmaticus
   5. Complications
      a. Asthma symptoms from histamine release after thiopental sodium injection, which are lessened by use of methohexital

## COMPARING LOCAL ANESTHETIC AGENTS

Local anesthetics prevent or relieve pain by blocking the generation and conduction of nerve impulses. Most can be administered by local infiltration or injection into the epidural or subarachnoid spaces of the spinal cord; each can be given by additional routes of administration that extend its spectrum of use.

Sensory function diminishes in the following predictable sequence: vasomotor paralysis causes skin vasodilation; loss of cold sensation is followed by a brief sense of warmth, then by a loss of both warmth and cold; pain sensation is blocked (slow pain sensation is diminished first, followed by fast pain sensation); light touch becomes dulled; and finally, proprioception and skeletal muscle tone are lost.

Recovery proceeds in the reverse order. Knowing this sequence will help the nurse ensure the patient's comfort as the anesthetic begins to take effect and make an appropriate assessment as the anesthetic effects begin to diminish. Remember that, after epidural spinal anesthesia, sympathetic and sensory activity do not necessarily return simultaneously.

| AGENT | ROUTE | NURSING CONSIDERATIONS |
|---|---|---|
| **Amides** | | |
| mepivacaine (Isocaine) | • Local infiltration<br>• Epidural anesthesia<br>• Peripheral nerve block | • Keep emergency drugs and equipment at hand during anesthetic administration.<br>• This drug is especially useful in elderly patients or those with cardiovascular disease because it does not contain epinephrine. |
| bupivacaine (Marcaine) | • Epidural anesthesia<br>• Local infiltration<br>• Peripheral nerve block<br>• Spinal anesthesia | • Keep drugs and equipment for resuscitation at hand during anesthetic administration.<br>• Anticipate frequent aspiration to avoid intravascular administration<br>• Prevent maternal hypotension in peripheral or epidural block by elevating the patient's legs and positioning her on her left side.<br>• Expect to see cautious use of an anesthetic with a vasoconstrictor in an elderly patient or a patient with cardiovascular disease.<br>• Liver disease may prolong the half-life of bupivacaine.<br>• Do not use a solution with preservatives for epidural or spinal block.<br>• Discard partially used vials of anesthetic without preservatives.<br>• The 0.75% bupivacaine solution is no longer recommended in obstetric anesthesia. |
| lidocaine (Xylocaine) | • Epidural anesthesia<br>• Local infiltration<br>• Peripheral nerve block<br>• Spinal anesthesia<br>• Topical anesthesia | • Liver disease may prolong the half-life of lidocaine.<br>• Use solutions with epinephrine cautiously in patients with cardiovascular disease.<br>• Keep drugs and equipment for resuscitation at hand during anesthetic administration.<br>*(continued)* |

**COMPARING LOCAL ANESTHETIC AGENTS** *continued*

| AGENT | ROUTE | NURSING CONSIDERATIONS |
|---|---|---|
| lidocaine (Xylocaine) *continued* | | • Administer lidocaine with caution in an elderly patient or a patient with large areas of broken skin or mucous membranes.<br>• After anesthetizing the mouth or pharynx with lidocaine, have the patient wait 1 hour before eating. |
| prilocaine (Citanest) | • Local infiltration<br>• Peripheral nerve blocks | • Same as for bupivacaine. |
| **Esters** | | |
| procaine (Novocain) | • Local infiltration<br>• Peripheral nerve block<br>• Spinal anesthesia | • Anticipate hypersensitivity testing before procaine administration.<br>• Procaine is contraindicated for a patient who is hypersensitive to any other ester anesthetic. |
| chloroprocaine (Nesacaine) | • Epidural anesthesia<br>• Local infiltration<br>• Peripheral nerve block | • Anticipate hypersensitivity testing before chloroprocaine administration.<br>• Chloroprocaine is contraindicated for a patient who is hypersensitive to any other ester anesthetic. |
| tetracaine (Pontocaine) | • Topical anesthesia | • Tetracaine is contraindicated for a patient who is allergic to procaine or PABA.<br>• Clean and dry the rectal area before applying tetracaine.<br>• Tetracaine is contraindicated for a patient with hypersensitivity to any other ester anesthetic. |
| cocaine | • Topical anesthesia | • Cocaine is contraindicated for a patient who is hypersensitive to any other ester anesthetic.<br>• Cocaine is used intraoperatively on oral, laryngeal, and nasal mucosa.<br>• Administer cocaine cautiously to a patient with hypertension, cardiovascular disease, or hyperthyroidism. |

    b. Hypotension and cardiovascular collapse from depression of the cardiovascular system (dose dependent)
    c. Tissue necrosis from extravascular infiltration
    d. Possible limb amputation if intra-arterial injection occurs
  6. Examples
    a. Thiopental sodium (Pentothal)
    b. Methohexital sodium (Brevital)

7. Nursing responsibilities
   a. Instruct the patient to take several deep breaths as he begins to lose consciousness, and tell him that a garlic taste just before losing consciousness is normal
   b. Have resuscitative equipment and emergency drugs available
   c. Administer methohexital sodium in dextrose 5% in water or normal saline solution because it is incompatible with lactated Ringer's solution or acid drug solutions, such as atropine
   d. Assess the patient for a red rash or flush across the chest from histamine release
   e. Check the patient's cardiopulmonary status and vital signs before, during, and after anesthesia
   f. Limit conversation and extraneous noise because hearing is the last sense to be lost before unconsciousness

C. **Narcotics**
   1. General information
      a. Are administered by intravenous or intramuscular injection as part of most general anesthetic techniques; several short-acting narcotics have been developed primarily for anesthetic use
      b. Can reduce the amount of inhalation anesthetic required by blunting the sympathetic response (increase in heart rate and blood pressure) to surgery and providing analgesia
      c. Can be used for anesthesia when given in high doses and combined with nitrous oxide, oxygen, and a neuromuscular blocking agent, a technique popularized in the 1970s
      d. Reduce plasma catecholamine, which can generate cardiac arrhythmias, and may cause pinpoint pupils
      e. Can be reversed by the narcotic antagonist naloxone
   2. Mechanism of action
      a. Stimulate opiate receptors in the brain and spinal cord
      b. Alter perception of and emotional response to pain
   3. Uses
      a. Perioperative analgesia (low doses)
      b. Anesthesia (high doses)
      c. Blunting the sympathetic response to endotracheal intubation
      d. Calming anxious patients
   4. Contraindications
      a. Allergy to drug
      b. Head injury (use cautiously)
   5. Complications
      a. Dose-dependent respiratory depression (anesthesia team must be prepared to ventilate the patient manually)
      b. Muscle rigidity from rapid administration (woody chest), relieved by administration of a neuromuscular blocking agent
      c. Bradycardia

      d. Nausea and vomiting

      e. Vasodilation and hypotension (morphine)

  6. Examples

      a. Fentanyl (Sublimaze)

      b. Sufentanil (Sufenta)

      c. Alfentanil (Alfenta)

      d. Morphine

      e. Meperidine (Demerol)

  7. Nursing responsibilities

      a. Check the availability of a narcotic antagonist, such as naloxone, before administering narcotics (naloxone reverses respiratory depression, which can cause hypoxia and death)

      b. Monitor respiratory status frequently, as indicated by the patient's level of responsiveness

      c. Caution the patient that itching commonly occurs after narcotic administration, especially when given intravenously

## D. Antianxiety agents

  1. General information

      a. Are commonly used in general anesthetic techniques and include benzodiazepines, butyrophenones, and phenothiazines

      b. Are usually administered intravenously but can be given intramuscularly in the operating room if the patient is agitated and an I.V. line has not been established

      c. Are given in titrated doses until onset of dysarthria (slurred speech) when administered in the operating room

      d. Cannot be reversed because no specific antagonist exists

      e. Induce amnesia in high doses, a sometimes undesirable effect that can distress the patient, and act as anticonvulsants by relaxing skeletal muscle and depressing nervous system structures (benzodiazepines)

      f. Cause pain on injection because of the solution's high alkalinity (diazepam); a water-soluble agent is significantly less painful to inject (midazolam)

      g. May have a second peak effect 6 to 8 hours after initial administration, causing the patient to return to drowsiness (diazepam)

      h. Cause sedation and relieve nausea (butyrophenones and phenothiazines)

      i. Have a long duration of action (12 to 24 hours) and produce sleepy, detached patients (droperidol)

      j. Can produce *neuroleptanalgesia* through a combination of narcotics and droperidol

  2. Mechanism of action

      a. Exhibit some degree of alpha-adrenergic blockade that may decrease blood pressure levels

      b. Interfere with interneuronal transmission at the spinal cord

      c. Interfere with central nervous system (CNS) transmission at certain receptors (phenothiazines and droperidol)

      d.  Inhibit chemoreceptor trigger zone in the medulla to act as an antiemetic

3.  Uses
   a.  Calm patient and allay anxiety
   b.  Induce amnesia (benzodiazepines)
   c.  Relieve nausea (butyrophenones, phenothiazines)
   d.  Diminish recall of unpleasant procedures (endotracheal intubation, endoscopy, cardioversion)
   e.  Sedate patient for brief procedures or those done under local or regional anesthesia

4.  Contraindications
   a.  Allergy to drug
   b.  Pregnancy (fetal malformations can occur when benzodiazepines are administered to a pregnant patient)
   c.  Parkinson's disease

5.  Complications
   a.  Exacerbation of Parkinson's disease or production of similar extrapyramidal symptoms (butyrophenones)
   b.  Paradoxic reaction of agitation and anxiety rather than sedation
   c.  Respiratory depression when benzodiazepines are combined with narcotics (midazolam has been associated with significant respiratory depression and death in patients, especially elderly and debilitated patients, who were not monitored closely)
   d.  Hypotonia and jaundice in breast-feeding infants (benzodiazepines are excreted in breast milk)
   e.  Hypotension, especially orthostatic hypotension postoperatively
   f.  Inner storm, in which patient appears calm and detached but postoperatively reports agitation and anxiety (droperidol)

6.  Examples
   a.  Benzodiazepines — midazolam (Versed), diazepam (Valium), lorazepam (Ativan)
   b.  Butyrophenones — droperidol (Inapsine)
   c.  Phenothiazines — hydroxyzine (Vistaril), promethazine (Phenergan)

7.  Nursing responsibilities
   a.  Seek out the source of the patient's anxiety, and remember that antianxiety agents are not substitutes for compassion or communication
   b.  Ensure that resuscitative equipment is at hand
   c.  Never give benzodiazepines to a woman who is or may be pregnant
   d.  Keep the environment quiet and professional; a patient who appears sedated may in fact be anxious
   e.  Instruct the patient not to get out of bed without assistance
   f.  Reassure and reorient the patient as necessary; amnesia can occur after benzodiazepine administration
   g.  Notify the physician immediately of extrapyramidal reactions to droperidol

**E. Dissociative anesthetic agent (ketamine)**
1. General information
   a. Is a nonbarbiturate, nonnarcotic anesthetic agent similar to the illegal drug phencyclidine (PCP) and given intravenously or intramuscularly for general anesthesia
   b. Produces profound analgesia in low doses and anesthesia in higher doses with a rapid onset of action, even after intramuscular injection
   c. May cause purposeless movements
   d. Cannot be reversed because no antagonist is available
   e. Can produce psychic side effects, such as hallucinations and nightmares, which are diminished by concurrent administration of diazepam
2. Mechanism of action
   a. Functionally dissociates the limbic and thalamocortical systems in the brain to produce intense analgesia and detached affect
   b. Stimulates cardiovascular and respiratory systems by central sympathetic stimulation innervation
3. Uses
   a. Analgesia (low dose)
   b. Anesthesia (high dose)
   c. Anesthesia or analgesia for burn patients (especially those with burns of the face and hands because airway manipulation and I.V. administration may be difficult)
   d. Anesthesia in trauma patients and some emergency obstetric patients who are hemorrhaging or in shock
4. Contraindications
   a. Allergy to drug
   b. Severe hypertension, ischemic heart disease, and increased intracranial pressure or stroke
   c. Intraocular surgery (diplopia, eye movements, and nystagmus may occur)
   d. History of psychiatric disorder
5. Complications
   a. Emergence reactions—hallucinations, nightmares, behavioral disturbances, and psychosis (incidence is as high as 12% and can occur hours or weeks after administration)
   b. Hypertension and tachycardia
   c. Increased intracranial pressure
6. Example: Ketamine (Ketalar)
7. Nursing responsibilities
   a. Plan nursing care around the drug's potential side effects; adequate monitoring must be balanced by the patient's need for minimal stimulation
   b. Dim lights, limit visitors, turn off the television, and speak softly
   c. Reassure and reorient the patient as needed for the first 24 hours or until the patient recovers from ketamine's effects

**F. Neuromuscular blocking agents**
1. General information
   a. Are part of many general anesthetic procedures and form the third element in the anesthesia triad — analgesia, amnesia, muscle relaxation
   b. Interfere with activity at the neuromuscular junction (where the terminal fibers of motor nerves meet the skeletal muscles)
   c. Cause muscle weakness or complete paralysis, depending on the dose injected
   d. Are commonly referred to as *muscle relaxants* but must not be confused with such relaxants as cyclobenzaprine (Flexeril) or carisoprodol (Soma), which are used for muscle strains or backaches
   e. Have no effect on pain or mental activity, and in most cases anesthetics to induce unconsciousness should be administered concurrently
   f. Are classified as *depolarizing* (mimic the action of acetylcholine at the neuromuscular junction, can cause involuntary muscle contractions [fasciculations] after I.V. injection, typically responsible for patient complaints of intense postoperative muscle soreness) or *nondepolarizing* (inhibit the action of acetylcholine at the neuromuscular junction)
   g. Are destroyed in the bloodstream by the enzyme pseudocholinesterase (depolarizing agents)
2. Mechanism of action
   a. Block transmission of electrical impulses from nerve to muscle, rendering the muscle weak or flaccid
   b. Eliminate and redistribute electrical charges at the neuromuscular junction by mimicking the neurotransmitter acetylcholine (depolarizing agents)
   c. Compete with acetylcholine for receptor sites at the neuromuscular junction and inhibit rather than mimic the action of acetylcholine (nondepolarizing agents)
3. Uses
   a. Balance anesthetic technique
   b. Facilitate endotracheal intubation and surgery by reducing muscle tone and resistance
   c. Improve manipulation of joints under anesthesia in orthopedic operations
   d. Relax muscles to prevent injury during electroconvulsive therapy under anesthesia (depolarizing agents)
   e. Prevent movement during surgery, especially in critically ill patients with compromised cardiovascular status who cannot tolerate the levels of anesthesia needed to prevent movement
   f. Prevent intubated patients from working against the mechanical ventilator
4. Contraindications
   a. Allergy to drug
   b. History or suspicion of malignant hyperthermia or low pseudocholinesterase levels (depolarizing agents)
5. Complications
   a. Triggering of malignant hyperthermia (depolarizing agents)

       b. Sudden hyperkalemia from release of potassium during depolarization leading to cardiac arrest; most common in burn and recent trauma patients (depolarizing agents)

       c. Postoperative myalgia from fasciculations (depolarizing agents)

       d. Histamine release and hypotension (nondepolarizing agents)

       e. Tachycardia (nondepolarizing agents)

       f. Unresponsiveness to manual ventilation after neuromuscular blockade

       g. Awareness of intraoperative events with inadequate anesthesia

    6. Examples

       a. Nondepolarizing agents — curare (Tubocurarine), metocurine (Metubine), pancuronium (Pavulon), vecuronium (Norcuron), atracurium (Tracrium)

       b. Depolarizing agent — succinylcholine (Anectine), commonly noted on chart as "sux" or "sch"

    7. Nursing responsibilities

       a. Never administer neuromuscular blocking agents unless all equipment (endotracheal tube, laryngoscope, ventilating bag and mask, oxygen, and suction) for maintaining respiration is at hand; hypoxia and death result if the patient is not ventilated

       b. Do not mistake neuromuscular blocking agents for muscle relaxants

       c. Be aware that the patient receiving neuromuscular blocking agents cannot speak or move but may still feel pain

       d. Choose words carefully when caring for trauma patients or critically ill patients in the operating room; they may tolerate only a minimal amount of anesthesia and receive neuromuscular blocking agents to facilitate surgery, leaving them conscious at times

       e. Consult the physician for an order for benzodiazepine tranquilizers and analgesics as necessary to help diminish patient recall

       f. Check whether succinylcholine was administered if a patient complains of postoperative muscle soreness, and reassure him that this normally subsides in 1 to 3 days

       g. Notify the surgeon and anesthesia team if muscle soreness does not resolve

**G. Reversal agents**

    1. General information

       a. Reverse narcotics and nondepolarizing blocking agents

       b. Do not reverse barbiturates, antianxiety agents, dissociative or inhalation agents, or the depolarizing blocking agent succinylcholine

    2. Mechanism of action

       a. Increase the amount of acetylcholine at the neuromuscular junction to reverse nondepolarizing blocking agents (anticholinesterase agents)

       b. Displace the narcotic from opiate receptors in the brain (narcotic antagonists and agonist-antagonists)

    3. Uses

       a. Reverse effects of nondepolarizing blocking agents to restore breathing and muscle tone

b. Reverse narcotic overdose
c. Reduce emergence delirium (agitation, combativeness)
4. Contraindications
   a. Allergy to drug
   b. Opiate dependency or acute opiate withdrawal
5. Complications
   a. Hypertension, tachycardia, and pulmonary edema after rapid reversal of narcotic analgesia
   b. Respiratory distress, hypoxia, and death from inadequate reversal of neuromuscular blocking agents
   c. Bradycardia and excessive secretions from anticholinesterase agents
6. Examples
   a. Neuromuscular blocking agent reversals — neostigmine (Prostigmin), pyridostigmine (Regonal), edrophonium (Tensilon)
   b. Anticholinergic drugs — glycopyrrolate (Robinul), atropine
   c. Narcotic agonist — naloxone (Narcan)
7. Nursing responsibilities
   a. Monitor the patient's respiratory status until arrival at the PACU, and request anesthesia team evaluation if breathing seems inadequate and patient is weak
   b. Administer oxygen in the PACU, and prepare to start mechanical ventilation if necessary to maintain breathing and oxygenation
   c. Reassure the patient to reduce anxiety from intubation and assume the role of patient advocate because an intubated patient cannot speak
   d. Do not extubate until the patient can sustain a head lift for 10 seconds and grip hands firmly (or until ordered; check agency policy)

**H. Inhalation agents**
1. General information
   a. Are inhaled via an endotracheal tube or mask placed over the face
   b. May be used in young children who cannot tolerate I.V. administration
2. Inhalation induction
   a. Liquid agents are heated to vapor by the anesthesia machine and delivered to the lungs in a carrier gas
   b. Carrier gases used in anesthesia include oxygen (always administered with any anesthetic), nitrous oxide (laughing gas, often used concurrently to provide analgesia and amnesia), and air
   c. The heart circulates the agent to the vital organs, and unconsciousness ensues when concentrations in the brain exceed a critical level
   d. Carrier gas and vapor are transported from the machine to the patient by the anesthesia breathing circuit, and a strong alkali, such as barium hydroxide lime, is placed in this circuit to absorb most of the carbon dioxide from the patient
   e. As surgery is completed, anesthetic concentrations are decreased and discontinued; the anesthetic diffuses from the brain into the bloodstream and is exhaled

    f. Consciousness returns in minutes or a few hours, depending on the duration of the anesthetic, other agents used, and the patient's condition

    g. Before ultrashort-acting barbiturates were available, patients inhaled the vapor until they lost consciousness, commonly causing excitement, struggling, coughing, and vomiting

    h. Injecting an ultrashort-acting barbiturate eliminates the excitement phase, and when the barbiturate's effect subsides, the inhalation agent has anesthetized the patient

3. Mechanism of action

    a. Exact mechanism unknown

    b. Believed to interrupt CNS transmission by depressing excitatory transmission in the cerebral cortex

4. Uses

    a. Produce unconsciousness during surgery

    b. Relax skeletal muscle

5. Contraindications

    a. Family history of malignant hyperthermia

    b. History of seizure disorder or renal disease (relative contraindication to enflurane because of nephrotoxicity and CNS irritation)

6. Complications

    a. Hypotension, shock, and cardiac arrest from overdosage (inhalation anesthetics depress blood pressure in a dose-dependent manner)

    b. Malignant hyperthermia

    c. Airway obstruction and hypoxia

    d. Postoperation shivering

    e. Postoperation nausea and vomiting

    f. Liver toxicity

7. Examples

    a. Isoflurane (Forane)

    b. Enflurane (Ethrane)

    c. Halothane (Fluothane)

8. Nursing responsibilities

    a. Ensure that the patient has not eaten for 8 hours before surgery to prevent aspiration

    b. Monitor the patient's vital signs frequently; assess adequacy, rate, and depth of patient's ventilations; and maintain a patent airway

    c. Assess the patient's level of consciousness, arousal, and orientation

    d. Exercise caution when giving additional analgesics before complete recovery from anesthesia; analgesic doses vary, depending on the residual anesthetic effect

    e. Inform the patient that psychomotor functions may be impaired for 24 hours or more

    f. Keep the patient warm with additional blankets to minimize shivering

## Points to Remember

Amides and esters are local anesthetic agents.

Barbiturates are injected intravenously to induce anesthesia.

Inhalation agents are used to maintain anesthesia after induction with ultrashort-acting barbiturates.

Narcotics, antianxiety agents, and neuromuscular blocking agents are integral to most general anesthetic procedures.

Recovery from ketamine anesthesia requires a balance between adequate patient monitoring and minimal stimulation.

## Glossary

**Acetylcholine** — neurotransmitter involved in transmitting nerve impulses at the neuromuscular junction

**Inhalation anesthetics** — volatile liquids heated to vapor and inhaled; carried by oxygen or oxygen-nitrous oxide mixture to maintain anesthesia

**Narcotics** — opiate analgesics used as adjuncts to anesthesia to relieve pain and anxiety and, in high doses, to produce anesthesia

**Neuroleptanalgesia** — anesthesia produced by combining a narcotic with the butyrophenone droperidol

**Neuromuscular blocking agents** — pharmacologic agents that block conduction of electrical impulses at the neuromuscular junction to produce muscle relaxation; facilitate intubation and surgery and require mechanical support of respiration

# Intraoperative Nursing

**Learning Objectives**

After studying this section, the reader should be able to:

- Identify the three zones of the surgical suite.

- Discuss types of instruments used in the operating room.

- Describe the purpose of sponge, instrument, and needle counts.

- Name two types of suture materials and their uses.

- Compare and contrast methods of maintaining hemostasis.

- Discuss equipment safety measures.

- Identify three aspects of the patient's condition that require routine monitoring.

- Describe the documentation necessary for perioperative events.

# VIII. Intraoperative Nursing

A. **Introduction**
  1. The intraoperative phase begins when the patient is placed on the surgical table and ends with transport to the postanesthesia care unit (PACU)
  2. All resources and team members are prepared before the patient enters the operating room (OR) to prevent unnecessary delays during surgery
  3. Information about the patient's and surgeon's needs is obtained from the medical record, surgery schedule, and surgeon's preference card
     a. The medical record provides information on specific patient requirements, such as adaptations that might be needed during surgery to accommodate a patient's disability
     b. The surgeon's preference card states preferred equipment, supplies, instruments, and patient position
  4. The circulating nurse provides direct patient care intraoperatively (see Appendix B, Nursing Process Applied to the Intraoperative Phase)

B. **Surgical suite**
  1. General information
     a. The surgical suite encompasses ORs and support areas, such as the preoperative holding area and the PACU
     b. An aseptic environment must be maintained to conduct surgical procedures
     c. The area can become a fire hazard because of the liberal use of oxygen and increasing use of paper disposable drapes
     d. Risk of microbial contamination is decreased through dress code and traffic flow procedures
  2. Suite design
     a. Preoperative holding area, usually located at the front of the surgical suite, receives patients from nursing units and provides a place for family members to wait with the patient until transport to the OR
     b. A central control desk serves as an information point for team members and visitors
     c. Design is such that patients transported to ORs do not encounter those transported to the PACU after surgery
     d. ORs open into the main corridor and a substerilizing room, which provides an area where instruments can be sterilized between procedures and may also contain scrub sinks for the surgical handscrub
     e. ORs are designed with one wall away from doorways and traffic, which is designated as the sterile field
  3. Physical requirements of ORs
     a. Temperature is usually maintained between 68° and 75° F (20° and 24° C) for comfort of sterile team members and inhibition of bacterial growth
     b. Neonates and infants require temperatures from 78.8° to 80.6° F (26° to 27° C) because they cannot regulate body temperature

    c. Humidity is maintained at a minimum of 50% to suppress static electricity, and incremental temperature adjustments must be made to avoid condensation that might drip onto sterile items

    d. Ventilation is provided by a controlled filtered system: air enters through vents in the central part of the ceiling and recirculates via floor vents on opposing walls (air exchange) to produce a downward flow

    e. At least 25 air exchanges per hour, five of which should be fresh air, are necessary

    f. Positive pressure is created inside so that outside air is prevented from entering the OR as personnel enter or exit

4. Traffic flow

    a. Traffic flow in the OR suite is determined by three zones (unrestricted, semirestricted, and restricted), which dictate who may enter and what they must wear

    b. *Unrestricted* zones (preoperative holding area, PACU, lounge, classrooms) have no attire restrictions, and family members can enter with the patient

    c. *Semirestricted* zones (corridors leading to ORs, central supply area, instrument processing area) require scrub apparel, hats, and shoe covers

    d. *Restricted* zones (ORs and substerilizing rooms) require scrub apparel, hats, shoe covers, and face masks

5. Dress code

    a. Only hospital-laundered scrubs, which are changed daily and when soiled, are worn in the OR suite

    b. Surgical scrubs are designed to decrease the possibility of bacterial penetration

    c. Shoe covers prevent tracking of substances from outside areas into the aseptic environment and are removed before leaving the OR suite to prevent transport of contaminants to other hospital areas

    d. High-filtration masks, which cover the mouth and nose, are worn in restricted zones to decrease the possibility of infection

    e. Jewelry must be covered or removed to prevent it from falling onto a sterile area or otherwise contaminating the room

    f. Nail polish is prohibited in restricted and semirestricted zones because it can harbor bacteria

6. Nursing responsibilities

    a. Be aware of the required attire for each zone

    b. Ensure that all OR visitors comply with traffic flow and dress code procedures

    c. Keep OR doors closed to maintain positive pressure inside the room, and minimize traffic to and from the OR to prevent pressure changes

## C. Instrumentation

1. General information

    a. Surgical instruments cut, clamp, hold, or retract tissue and are categorized according to function

    b. Most surgical instruments are made of surgical stainless steel, and their names vary according to manufacturer, surgeon, and region (see *Surgical instruments,* pages 74 to 77)

    c. Instrument size varies according to the depth of the surgical site, determined by the type of procedure or size of the patient

    d. Instrument sets are designed for specific procedures

2. Cutting instruments (sharps)

    a. Used for cutting tissue, suture material, and dressings

    b. Designed for dissection of delicate tissue (Metzenbaum scissors), cutting dressings or tough tissue such as fascia (Mayo scissors), or cutting skin and deep tissues (scalpels)

3. Clamping instruments

    a. Control bleeding but can also hold or retract tissue; examples are hemostats and Kelly clamps

    b. Obstruct the lumen of a vessel before or after dissection (clamp tips)

    c. Vary in tip size, depending on the size of the vessel being clamped

4. Holding (grasping) instruments

    a. Hold sutures or tissue being manipulated, sutured, or dissected; examples are needle holders, tissue forceps, Allis clamps, Oschner clamps, and Babcock clamps

    b. Vary in tip size, depending on the type of tissue being held; a sharp or teethed tip is used on tough tissues or those to be resected, and an atraumatic tip is used for delicate tissues

5. Retracting instruments

    a. Are designed to pull tissue away to expose the surgical site; examples are Army-Navy, Deaver, Ribbon, Richardson, glass, and rake

    b. Have a locking mechanism to hold the retractor open and maintain exposure (self-retaining retractors) or are held in place by the surgeon or surgical assistant (hand-held retractors)

6. Nursing responsibilities

    a. Be familiar with the types of instruments and their uses, and confirm that they are in good working condition

    b. Inspect instruments containing several parts before handing to the surgeon and when returned to verify that no parts have been left inside the patient

    c. Exercise care when cleaning and preparing surgical instruments for use because they are expensive to replace

## D. Counts

1. General information

    a. Counts ensure patient safety and prevent instrument loss through inventory of items during surgery

    b. Sponges, instruments, suture needles, hypodermic needles, and anything else on the sterile field that could be retained in the wound are counted

    c. Items used within the surgical wound should be detectable by X-rays

*(Text continues on page 77.)*

# SURGICAL INSTRUMENTS

## CUTTING INSTRUMENTS

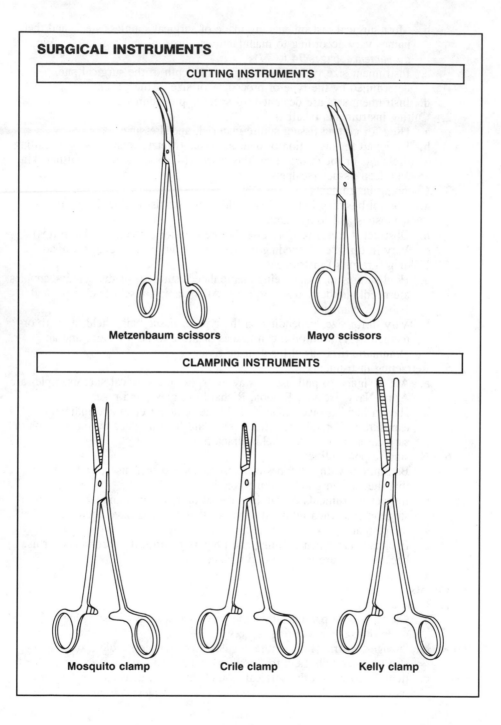

Metzenbaum scissors          Mayo scissors

## CLAMPING INSTRUMENTS

Mosquito clamp          Crile clamp          Kelly clamp

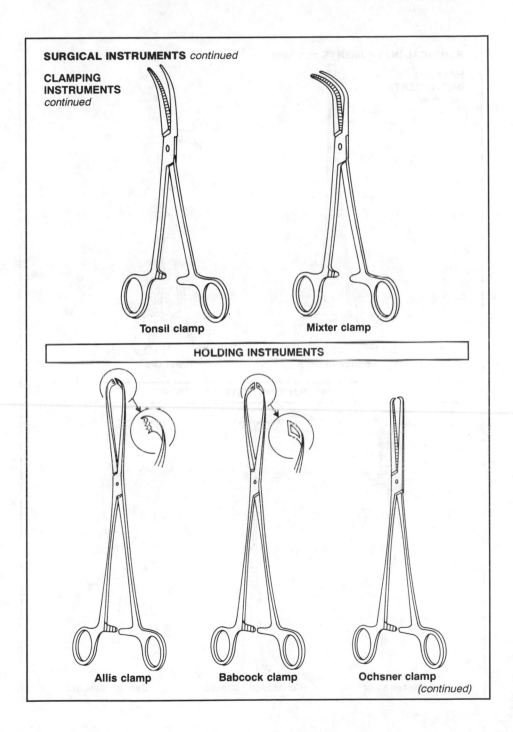

**SURGICAL INSTRUMENTS** *continued*

**CLAMPING INSTRUMENTS**
*continued*

Tonsil clamp

Mixter clamp

**HOLDING INSTRUMENTS**

Allis clamp

Babcock clamp

Ochsner clamp

*(continued)*

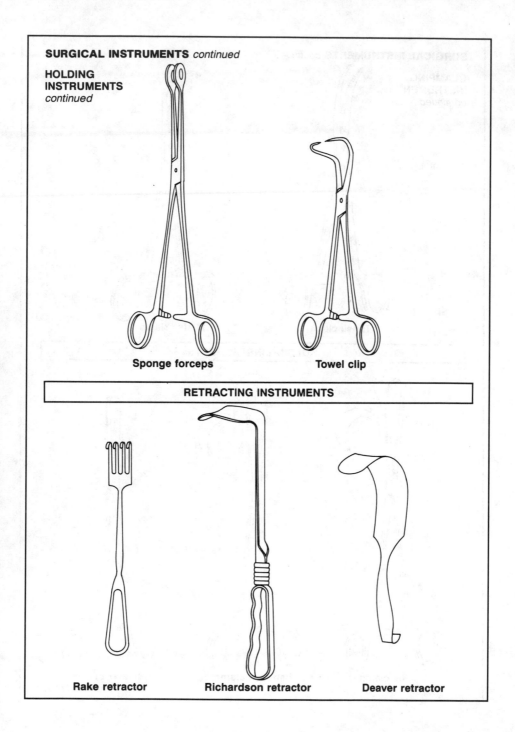

**SURGICAL INSTRUMENTS** *continued*

**HOLDING INSTRUMENTS**
*continued*

Sponge forceps

Towel clip

**RETRACTING INSTRUMENTS**

Rake retractor

Richardson retractor

Deaver retractor

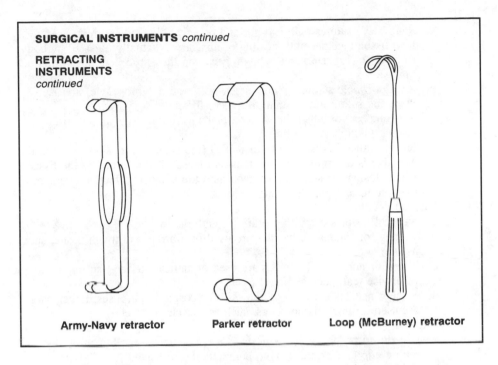

SURGICAL INSTRUMENTS *continued*

RETRACTING
INSTRUMENTS
*continued*

**Army-Navy retractor**          **Parker retractor**          **Loop (McBurney) retractor**

2. Count procedure
   a. At least three counts are performed—before the incision is made, before closing the first tissue layer, and during closing of the last tissue layer
   b. The circulating nurse counts all items with the scrub nurse, records the initial count on the clinical record, and notes items obtained during the procedure
   c. Once all items are counted, the wound is closed and counts are documented as correct
   d. Any discrepancies in the count are reported to the surgeon, who stops the closing procedure to search for the missing item
   e. If the item cannot be found by reexploring the wound, an X-ray is taken to determine if the item has been retained
3. Nursing responsibilities
   a. Ensure accurate count by watching items as they are counted
   b. Make notations on the count sheet when items are added to the field

**E. Sutures, surgical needles, and clips**
   1. General information
      a. Are used for blood vessel ligation (suture ties) and wound closure
      b. Can be freehand or attached to a needle (sutures)

2. Sutures
   a. *Absorbable* sutures (surgical gut and polyglycolic acid sutures), used to hold tissue together until healing occurs, are eventually digested by body enzymes or broken down by hydrolysis and then absorbed; absorption time varies
   b. *Nonabsorbable* sutures (nylon, steel, silk, and polypropylene) are used when the suture must remain in place (for example, vascular anastomoses) or when the surgeon plans to remove the sutures after healing (skin closure sutures)
   c. Sutures range in diameter from #10.0 (the smallest) to #5 (the largest)
   d. The size is determined by the tension placed on the suture by the tissues; when closing the skin, the surgeon uses the smallest effective diameter possible to minimize scarring
3. Surgical needles
   a. Surgical needles carry the suture through tissue
   b. Cutting, or traumatic, needles are used on fibrous and tough tissue, such as skin
   c. Taper, or noncutting, needles are used on delicate tissue that might otherwise tear, such as bowel tissue
   d. Smaller needles are used on the skin for cosmetic purposes; larger ones are used on thick tissue layers, such as muscle or fascia
4. Clips
   a. Clips used primarily for hemostasis are attached to the lumen of vessels with a clip applier and remain permanently in place
   b. Clips used for wound closure are applied with a clip applier and usually removed when tissue is repaired
   c. Stainless steel or titanium clips are available
5. Nursing responsibilities
   a. Refer to the surgeon's preference card for selection of suture and needle types
   b. Carefully check labels and needles to prevent possible tissue damage from use of an inappropriate needle or suture
   c. Ensure that clip appliers have been correctly loaded to prevent possible damage from misfired instrument or misplaced clip
   d. Count instruments, needles, and sponges used during surgery

F. **Hemostasis**
   1. General information
      a. Most surgical procedures result in some blood loss, which is minimized by using methods of hemostasis
      b. Many patients are reluctant to receive blood products because of the possibility of disease transmission
   2. Natural hemostasis
      a. Natural hemostasis is the body's response to blood vessel injury
      b. When the integrity of the vessel lumen is disrupted, platelets adhere to the injured area, forming a platelet plug

      c. As platelets break down, they release thromboplastin, which unites with prothrombin and calcium ions in the blood to form thrombin

      d. Thrombin joins with the blood plasma fibrinogen to form fibrin, the basic structure of the blood clot

      e. Although natural hemostasis is necessary to control bleeding, additional measures are needed to ensure adequate control

  3. Artificial hemostasis

      a. To initiate and maintain hemostasis artificially, the surgical team places pressure on bleeding vessels to stop blood flow long enough for a clot to form or until the surgeon can arrest bleeding by other means

      b. Once the lumen has been occluded by a clamp, the surgeon or assistant applies a suture ligature or metal clip to obstruct blood flow permanently

      c. Topical agents (gelatin sponges, thrombin, oxidized cellulose) can accelerate or promote clot formation and are effective in areas oozing from capillary bleeding

      d. A cautery, used to control bleeding in small blood vessels, provides a high-frequency electrical current that coagulates blood

  4. Nursing responsibilities

      a. Ensure that appropriate supplies and equipment for hemostasis are available

      b. Check labels of topical agents before use, and check cords and wiring of cautery to minimize the possibility of sparking, which could start a fire in the presence of oxygen

      c. Apply dispersive, or grounding, pads for the cautery to areas that readily conduct electrical current, and inspect the skin for burns after removing the pad

      d. Ask the surgeon for the specific setting of the electric cautery unit to be used, and ensure that it has been set properly

      e. Discontinue use of the cautery unit if the alarm sounds or equipment malfunctions; indications of malfunction are muscle twitching during equipment activation and unexplained loss of power that requires higher-than-usual settings to accomplish coagulation

      f. Note the equipment number of the cautery unit so that the unit can be traced if a burn is detected later

      g. Explain to the patient measures taken to prevent bloodborne infection

## G. Equipment safety

  1. General information

      a. Electrical and pneumatic components of surgical equipment are potentially hazardous if not carefully inspected and operated

      b. The risk of injury is increased because an unconscious or heavily sedated patient cannot feel the injury

      c. Oxygen used to ventilate the patient is a potential hazard because it supports combustion

2. Electrical equipment
   a. All electrical equipment can short out if the wiring is faulty and must be inspected before use to ensure patient safety
   b. Warming blankets and lamps can burn the patient if not adequately padded or closely monitored to control temperature
   c. Lasers can cause thermal burns to the skin, tissues, and eyes of the patient or team members if inadvertently activated, used near flammable materials, or deflected in another direction by reflective instruments
   d. When lasers are used, an additional nurse is assigned to operate the controls
   e. Cauteries can burn if the return dispersive electrode is not properly placed on the patient, the unit is inappropriately activated, or the setting is too high
   f. Defibrillators can cause injury if improperly operated, especially in the presence of sodium chloride, a commonly used irrigation solution capable of carrying an electrical current
3. Pneumatic equipment
   a. Improperly assembled drills and saws can cause substantial tissue damage
   b. Tourniquets used to control bleeding can cause irreversible ischemic damage if applied too tightly or left in place too long
4. Nursing responsibilities
   a. Check cords and controls of all electrical equipment immediately before use, and set laser to the inactive mode when not in use
   b. Ensure that equipment is properly maintained by the biomedical department
   c. Check the settings and monitor the patient's skin for signs of thermal damage when using warming units, and place padding on pressure areas in contact with warming blankets; monitor the core temperature with rectal or esophageal temperature probes
   d. Protect the team members' and patient's eyes with wave-specific goggles or eye patches, and ensure that instruments are dulled or ebonized to prevent laser beam reflection
   e. Use nonflammable endotracheal tubes and low concentrations of oxygen for ventilation if the surgical site is in or near the airway
   f. Place signs on doors indicating laser use to prevent others from entering without eye protection, and cover windows to protect persons outside the room
   g. Have fire extinguishers available
   h. Be sure OR personnel operating potentially dangerous equipment are properly trained, and document ongoing individual preparation in personnel files

## H. Routine monitoring
1. General information
   a. The circulating nurse works closely with other team members to monitor the patient's general condition

    b. The circulating nurse is responsible for ensuring compliance with OR rules and regulations designed to protect the patient from injury, infection, and invasion of privacy

  2. Urine output

    a. Bladder catheterization is usually performed for pelvic procedures to prevent distention from obstructing the surgical site or from laceration during tissue resection

    b. Blood in the urine indicates possible laceration of the bladder or ureters

    c. Urine output is monitored closely during critical procedures because decreased output or absence of urine may indicate inadequate tissue perfusion

  3. Blood loss

    a. Blood loss varies according to type and length of procedure, the patient's clotting ability and blood pressure, and the surgeon's ability to maintain hemostasis

    b. Blood suctioned from the surgical site is collected in graduated containers and measured; blood absorbed by surgical sponges is measured by weighing the sponges

  4. Temperature

    a. The patient's temperature should be monitored throughout the procedure

    b. Exposed body cavities, excessively cool environment, use of cool inspired gases, and central nervous system effects of anesthesia increase the risk of hypothermia

  5. Traffic flow

    a. The circulating nurse observes all team members for breaks in aseptic technique and discourages persons from entering or leaving the OR unnecessarily

    b. Excessive traffic increases the likelihood of stirring dust that could contaminate the surgical wound

    c. Unauthorized observers are not allowed in the OR

  6. Nursing responsibilities

    a. Measure urine output every 30 to 60 minutes as indicated, calculate blood loss, and report these results to the anesthesia team

    b. Prevent hypothermia by warming irrigation and I.V. fluids, placing the patient on a warming blanket, keeping the patient covered at all times, and maintaining a comfortable room temperature when possible

    c. Adjust room temperature or warming blanket settings to maintain the patient's temperature within normal limits

    d. Address and resolve breaks in aseptic technique

## I. Family support

  1. General information

    a. Separation during the intraoperative phase produces anxiety for the patient and family members

    b. Frequent communication with the family during the procedure alleviates anxiety associated with separation and loss of control

    c. Surgical team members communicate with others on the health-care team in the holding area, who relay information to the family; when the procedure is completed, the surgeon and other team members speak with the family directly

  2. Nursing responsibilities
    a. Meet the patient's significant other in the holding area, and discuss the procedure for calling the family during the intraoperative phase
    b. Call family members once the procedure is under way and every hour after that until the patient is transported to the PACU
    c. Report the patient's general condition, and explain that the surgeon will provide details after the procedure has been completed

**J. Documentation**
  1. Documentation by the circulating nurse provides a written account of OR events immediately before surgery, when critical information is verified and assessments made
  2. The surgical clinical record serves as a legal account of the procedure and provides valuable information to the postoperative nursing staff
  3. The preoperative assessment in the holding area, a necessary duplication of information already obtained by the preoperative nurse, consists of:
    a. Confirming patient identification and nothing-by-mouth status and notifying anesthesia team of any deviations from the order
    b. Verifying allergies on the chart with the patient and ensuring that all prosthetic devices, hair pins, and underclothing have been removed
    c. Checking, completing, and noting preoperative orders on the chart
    d. Reviewing the record for informed consent documents, history and physical, anesthesia evaluation, required laboratory work, and blood type and crossmatch, when applicable
  4. The circulating nurse documents the following intraoperative events:
    a. Skin condition for existing infection, irritation, and rashes, providing baseline data for later evaluation
    b. Arrival time in the surgical suite, incision time, time of wound closure, and departure time
    c. Names of all participants and their status
    d. Preoperative and postoperative diagnoses
    e. Location, size, and type of catheters, packings, and drains; type and amount of drainage or output
    f. Manufacturer, size, lot, and serial number of surgical implants
    g. Location of cautery return dispersive pad and skin condition
    h. Use, location, and settings of tourniquet
    i. Position of patient and supports used
    j. Sponge, needle, and instrument counts
    k. All nursing procedures and evaluation of nursing actions

5. The circulating nurse should also document any *unusual occurrence* — an incident or complication not part of a normal procedure
   a. Examples include cardiac or respiratory arrest; loss of a sponge, needle, or instrument; medication errors; adverse reaction to medications or blood products; and injuries related to positioning, equipment, or team members
   b. A copy of the medical record and an incident report are filed, allowing the risk management department to take appropriate actions to resolve the incident
   c. The circulating nurse collaborates with other team members to ensure complete documentation of the events
6. Nursing responsibilities
   a. Maintain neat, clean, and legible clinical records, and write all entries in ink
   b. Verify preoperative assessment information and titles, first names, and last names of all team members on the chart
   c. Rather than erase or cover a mistake with correction fluid, draw a single line through it, write "error," and sign the record; if a record must be recopied, staple the original to the new page
   d. Ensure that recorded data accurately reflect perioperative events
   e. Note unusual occurrences and describe events and the patient's condition before, during, and after the incident in detail

## Points to Remember

The design and maintenance of the surgical suite provide a safe environment for the patient to undergo surgery.

The surgical suite is divided into unrestricted, semirestricted, and restricted zones; semirestricted and restricted areas have specific attire requirements.

Use of oxygen in the operating room supports combustion and poses a fire hazard.

Surgical instruments are used for cutting, clamping, holding, and retracting tissues.

All items used in the surgical site must be counted before the surgeon closes the wound.

Because lasers significantly increase the likelihood of burns and fires, strict adherence to safety precautions is mandatory.

Frequent communication and collaboration among team members is essential when monitoring a patient's overall condition.

The surgical clinical record provides a written account of OR events to promote continuity of care.

## Glossary

**Laceration** — tearing of tissue

**Preoperative holding area** — place from which the patient is admitted to the OR and where requirements such as laboratory results, consent forms, and preoperative orders receive final confirmation

**Surgical scrub attire** — clothing made of fabric that meets or exceeds the National Fire Protection Association's "Standard for the Use of Inhalation Anesthetics"

# Intraoperative Positioning

**Learning Objectives**
After studying this section, the reader should be able to:

● Identify the most commonly used surgical positions.

● Describe the effects of positioning on major body systems.

● Provide examples of surgical procedures for which each position is used.

● Discuss nursing responsibilities to prevent patient injury in each position.

## IX. Intraoperative Positioning

### A. Introduction

1. A proper intraoperative position meets these criteria:
   a. Respiratory function uncompromised
   b. Adequate circulation maintained
   c. Nerves uncompressed
   d. Body weight distributed evenly
   e. Operation site accessible and adequately exposed
   f. Anesthetic administration unimpeded
   g. Postoperation discomfort minimized
   h. Patient characteristics considered
2. Various body systems that can be adversely affected during positioning as a result of anesthesia and immobility include:
   a. Integumentary system—sustained pressure on bony prominences (pressure points) can result in inadequate circulation that may lead to irreversible tissue necrosis; mechanical obstruction of blood flow (for example, by a safety strap applied too tightly) has similar effects (see *Positions and their possible pressure points,* pages 90 and 91)
   b. Circulatory system—general and regional anesthesia can produce profound vasodilation, which may lead to deep venous stasis of the lower extremities, formation of pulmonary emboli, and decreased oxygenated blood flow to the heart, brain, kidneys, and liver
   c. Respiratory system—compromised respiratory function from impaired diaphragmatic movement caused by hemidiaphragm pressure or impaired chest expansion caused by positive external pressure from improper support of the chest wall; improper patient positioning, especially during prolonged procedures, can cause decreased air exchange and impaired respiratory function, leading to atelectasis and decreased oxygenation
   d. Musculoskeletal system—absence of pain and pressure receptors, which normally prevent overstretching and hyperextension of muscle and tendon groups, expose the unconscious patient to risk of injury
   e. Nervous system—irreversible nerve damage resulting in sensory and motor loss can result from mechanical obstruction of blood flow to a nerve or nerve group and typically occurs because of inadequate pressure point padding
3. General nursing responsibilities include the following:
   a. Consult the anesthetist about any limitations or restrictions before moving a patient
   b. To prevent injury, move the patient slowly and gently, and never abduct the patient's arms more than 90 degrees or cross the patient's legs
   c. To prevent pressure sores from developing, pad body surface areas and all equipment, such as shoulder braces, used to position the patient
   d. To avoid electrical hazards, do not let the patient's body touch any metal table part

e.  Expose only the area necessary for surgery, to maintain the patient's privacy, and verify proper site exposure
f.  Ensure that equipment, such as a Mayo tray, does not put pressure on the patient's legs
g.  Ask for help when lifting the patient into position
h.  Document patient position, areas padded, assessment of pressure points, and measures taken to prevent injury

**B.  Supine position**
1.  General information
   a.  The patient is placed on his back, with arms tucked at the sides or extended on padded armboards
   b.  Most surgical procedures employ this position
   c.  Patients to be positioned otherwise usually undergo anesthesia in the supine position and are moved only after the airway is secured
   d.  Potential pressure points include occipital area, scapulae, thoracic vertebrae, olecranon (elbow), sacrum, coccyx, and calcaneous (heel)
2.  Indications
   a.  Abdominal procedures — hernia repair, cholecystectomy, abdominal aortic aneurysm repair, appendectomy
   b.  Head and neck procedures requiring an anterior approach — carotid endarterectomy, cervical fusion, thyroidectomy, frontal and temporal craniotomy, facial procedures
   c.  Arm and leg procedures — shoulder manipulations and reductions, open and closed reductions of the arms and legs, bunionectomy, peripheral vascular procedures, reconstructive procedures such as skin grafting
   d.  Breast procedures — mastectomy, biopsy, augmentation, reduction
3.  Nursing responsibilities
   a.  Maintain proper body alignment to prevent undue strain and pressure on muscles, nerves, and joints
   b.  Slowly and cautiously manipulate extremities to avoid overstretching and hyperextension; whenever resistance is met during manipulation, notify the surgeon before additional movement
   c.  Do not allow any body part to contact metal portions of or extend beyond the table to prevent external compression of nerves
   d.  Keep the patient's legs uncrossed to avoid obstruction of blood flow, and pad armboards to prevent nerve damage
   e.  Tuck the patient's arms at sides in a manner that maintains normal anatomic alignment; check capillary refill time after positioning to ensure adequate circulation
   f.  Secure the patient to the operating room table at all times, but apply safety straps loosely across the thighs so blood flow is not compromised

### C. Trendelenburg's position
1. General information
   a. In Trendelenburg's position, a modification of the supine position, the head of the table is lower than the foot
   b. This position allows increased blood flow to the upper body but can result in possible cerebral edema from prolonged positioning
   c. Trendelenburg's position results in an upward shifting of abdominal viscera to allow better visualization of pelvic structures
   d. Potential pressure points are similar to those for the supine position
2. Indications
   a. Pelvic procedures performed through the abdominal wall—abdominal hysterectomy, ovarian procedures, bladder procedures
   b. Diminished cerebral blood flow, such as in profound hypotension, hypovolemic shock, and cardiac arrest
3. Nursing responsibilities
   a. Adjust instrument tables to prevent the patient's feet from contacting them
   b. Use padded shoulder braces to stabilize a patient placed in an extreme position
   c. Work with other perioperative team members in limiting the time the patient remains in this position to prevent cerebral edema

### D. Sitting position
1. General information
   a. The back of the table is elevated to a vertical plane, knees are flexed, and arms are secured on a pillow across the abdomen
   b. The sitting position allows access to the posterior cervical area and posterior cranium
   c. The sitting position lowers arterial and venous pressure in the head and neck in relation to pressures of the heart, predisposing the patient to air embolism
   d. Potential pressure points include the scapulae, ischial tuberosities, back of the knee, and calcaneous
2. Indications
   a. Procedures of the cervical spine—posterior cervical laminectomy, removal of tumors of the posterior spine
   b. Procedures of the posterior and lateral cranium—posterior fossa craniotomy, temporal craniotomy, ventriculography
3. Nursing responsibilities
   a. Before flexing the table, be sure that the patient's hands are not near the breaks of the table to prevent injury to the fingers
   b. Apply antiembolism stockings to the legs to reduce venous pooling
   c. Adequately support the head, neck, shoulders, and trunk to prevent hyperflexion and hyperextension injuries of the spinal column
   d. Secure the patient to the table; after flexion, which increases the tension of the safety strap across the thighs, loosen the strap

e. If air embolism occurs, immediately return the patient to the supine position so that the surgical team can initiate appropriate resuscitative measures

## E. Lithotomy position
1. General information
   a. The lithotomy position is a modification of the supine position, with legs elevated, abducted, and supported in stirrups attached to the table
   b. After anesthesia induction, legs are slowly raised and placed in ankle or knee stirrups; the bottom section of the table is lowered to allow access to the perineal area
   c. Arms must be out to the side or secured across the abdomen to prevent the fingers from resting in the table break
   d. With the patient's legs raised, 500 to 800 ml of blood is diverted from lower extremities to the visceral area, masking effects of hypovolemia or resulting in profound hypotension in patients unable to compensate for rapid shifting of blood volume when legs are lowered
   e. Potential pressure points are similar to those for the supine position, except the calcaneous
2. Indications
   a. Vaginal procedures — vaginal hysterectomy, dilatation and curettage, cervical biopsy
   b. Rectal procedures — hemorrhoidectomy, sigmoidoscopy, repair of anal fistula
   c. Radical resections of the groin, vulva, and rectal areas
3. Nursing responsibilities
   a. Pad areas contacting metal portions of the stirrups to prevent external compression of nerves
   b. Do not allow the patient's hips to extend beyond the table to prevent strain on lumbosacral muscles from inadequate support of lower back
   c. Lower and raise both legs simultaneously (to prevent possible hip dislocation or muscle strain) and slowly (to allow the body to adjust to shifting blood volume)
   d. Apply antiembolism stockings for lengthy procedures to reduce venous stasis

## F. Lateral position
1. General information
   a. The patient lies on the unaffected side to expose the lateral chest wall or flank with a pillow between his legs; bottom leg is flexed and top leg remains straight
   b. Another pillow under the head maintains spinal column alignment, and a chest roll placed under the axilla promotes lung expansion
   c. The patient is moved into the lateral position after anesthesia induction

## POSITIONS AND THEIR POSSIBLE PRESSURE POINTS

The patient's body weight should be equally distributed on a surgical table. Proper padding of the bony prominences (pressure points) ensures adequate body weight distribution. This chart describes possible pressure points that the nurse should pad when the patient is placed in a specific position.

| POSITION | POSSIBLE PRESSURE POINTS |
|---|---|
| Supine 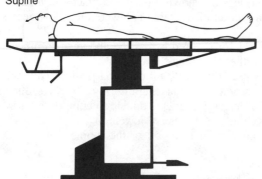 | • Occipital area<br>• Scapulae<br>• Thoracic vertebrae<br>• Olecranon<br>• Sacrum<br>• Coccyx<br>• Calcaneous |
| Trendelenburg's 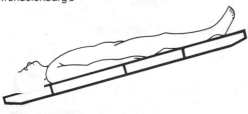 | • Same as for supine |
| Sitting 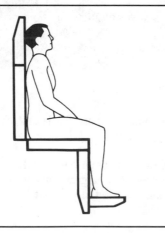 | • Scapulae<br>• Ischial tuberosities<br>• Back of knee<br>• Calcaneous |

**POSITIONS AND THEIR POSSIBLE PRESSURE POINTS** *continued*

| POSITION | POSSIBLE PRESSURE POINTS |
|---|---|
| Lithotomy 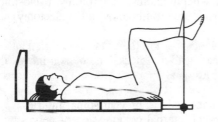 | ● Same as for supine, except for calcaneous |
| Lateral 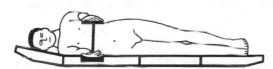 | ● Between legs, ankles, and feet<br>● Ear<br>● Acromion process<br>● Ribs<br>● Ilium<br>● Greater trochanter<br>● Medial and lateral condyles<br>● Maleolus |
| Prone 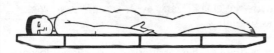 | ● Cheek<br>● Eyes<br>● Ears<br>● Acromion process<br>● Patella<br>● Toes<br>● Breasts (in women)<br>● Genitalia (in men) |
| Prone *(Jackknife)* 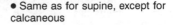 | ● Same as for prone |

    d. Potential pressure points include the legs, ankles, feet, ear, acromion process, ribs, iliac crest, greater trochanter, medial and lateral condyles, and maleolus

2. Indications
    a. Thoracotomy — resection, lobectomy, repair of descending aortic aneurysm
    b. Kidney and ureter procedures — nephrectomy, nephrotomy, pyelostomy, pyelolithotomy, nephrolithotomy, ureterolithotomy, adrenalectomy

3. Nursing responsibilities
    a. Use a minimum of four people to position the anesthetized patient; the anesthetist controls the patient's head and neck, one person moves the lower extremities, one person lifts and supports the shoulders and chest, and one controls the pelvis
    b. Conduct all movements simultaneously to prevent spinal injuries
    c. Pad all pressure points to prevent internal compression of nerves by bony prominences
    d. Secure the patient to the table with a safety strap or adhesive tape across the pelvis
    e. To prevent falls, ensure that adequate personnel are immediately available to place the patient in the supine position when surgery is completed

## G. Prone position
1. General information
    a. The patient is placed face down; flexion of the table at the hips creates the jackknife position
    b. Anesthesia is induced on the stretcher with the patient supine; once airway is secured, stretcher is aligned with surgical bed and the patient is rolled onto the table
    c. Lung expansion is considerably impaired if rolls are not placed anteriorly from the shoulders to the pelvis to lift chest off the bed
    d. Potential pressure points are the cheek, ears, eyes, acromion process, patella, toes, breasts, and genitalia

2. Indications
    a. Procedures of the rectum and anus — hemorrhoidectomy, sigmoidoscopy, anal fistula repair
    b. Procedures of the spine — lumbar laminectomy, lumbar fusion, removal of thoracic tumors, decompression of the spinal column

3. Nursing responsibilities
    a. Exercise caution when moving the patient from the stretcher onto the surgical table, and make sure that the stretcher and table are locked

b.  Use a minimum of four people to move the patient; one to support and move the head, one to support and move the lower body, one to support and move the torso, and one to control the body as it is rolled onto the table

c.  Avoid placing pressure on the patient's eyes to prevent injury

d.  Pad pressure points appropriately to avoid tissue and nerve damage from inadequate blood supply caused by obstruction of blood flow

## Points to Remember

Positioning the patient is a responsibility shared by all perioperative team members.

Mechanical obstruction of blood flow can cause irreversible tissue damage.

Patients must be secured to the surgical table at all times.

Whenever the surgical table is flexed, the nurse must ensure that the patient's fingers are not resting in the table break.

When repositioning an anesthetized patient, the anesthetist initiates the move and controls the patient's head and neck.

## Glossary

**Aneurysm** — abnormal dilation of a portion of a blood vessel, usually the result of atherosclerosis, infection, or trauma

**Atelectasis** — collapse of all or part of a lung

**Capillary refill time** — method of assessing circulation; refill can be tested by pressing the fingernail to produce blanching and observing the time it takes for return of color; sluggish return is associated with inadequate circulation

**Embolism** — intravascular movement of an object to another area where it obstructs or impedes blood flow; examples are air bubbles and blood clots

**Venous stasis** — pooling of blood in the venous system, usually in the lower extremities

# Intraoperative Complications

**Learning Objectives**

After studying this section, the reader should be able to:

- List the most common intraoperative complications and identify their causes.

- Describe the potential consequences of intraoperative complications.

- Discuss nursing responsibilities for each complication.

## X. Intraoperative Complications

### A. Introduction

1. Complications during the intraoperative phase are rare but can occur suddenly and cause serious injury or death
2. Surgery and anesthesia place the patient at risk even under ideal conditions
3. Many intraoperative complications, such as hemorrhage, cardiac arrhythmias, and cardiac arrest, can also occur postoperatively
4. Nursing actions during an intraoperative emergency can make a difference in the patient's outcome

### B. Difficult intubation

1. General information
   a. Intubation is the placement of a flexible breathing device, called an endotracheal tube, through the mouth or nose and into the larynx and trachea to maintain a patent airway
   b. A patient with a long, slender neck and full range of motion (ROM) of the head and neck and temporomandibular joint (TMJ) is usually easy to intubate
   c. Difficult intubation can be anticipated in some cases but may be unexpected in others
2. Types of intubation
   a. Direct—under direct vision with a laryngoscope, which comes in various sizes and typically consists of a handle with a lighted curved or straight blade
   b. Blind—by listening for breath sounds through the tube
   c. Fiberoptic—with the aid of a fiberoptic endoscope
   d. Retrograde—by passing a catheter through the trachea into the mouth, then guiding the tube over it
   e. Digital—by palpating the airway structures with the fingers (rarely used)
3. Causes
   a. Short, thick neck—epiglottis may be anteriorly placed and difficult to see
   b. Receding mandible—structures difficult to see
   c. Cervical traction or neck injury—limits manipulation of head-neck joint and minimizes visual exposure
   d. Degenerative joint disease in neck
   e. Large breasts and edematous airway structures in pregnant patients, especially at term
   f. Limited ROM of head and neck or TMJ
4. Treatment by anesthesia team
   a. Establish oxygen flow to the patient's lungs
   b. Continue mask ventilation to ensure oxygen flow; if oxygen cannot be moved into the lungs with positive pressure from mask ventilation, seek alternative delivery methods

    c. Perform cricothyrotomy when mask ventilation fails (the membrane between the thyroid and cricoid cartilages in the neck is punctured, and a small tube is inserted and connected to the oxygen source)

    d. Perform emergency tracheotomy if necessary

  5. Nursing responsibilities

    a. Keep in mind that surgery should not begin until the airway is secure

    b. Know the location of tracheotomy trays before starting any surgical procedure

    c. Be ready to assist the anesthesia team with suctioning, handing instruments, securing supplies, and applying cricoid pressure

    d. Notify the family of the complication if the situation warrants it and the physician in charge approves

## C. Arrhythmias

  1. General information

    a. Arrhythmias are aberrant heart rhythms that can be worsened by stress-induced catecholamine release from anxiety, noxious stimulation, laryngoscopy, or surgical stimulation

    b. Sinus arrhythmia and occasional premature ventricular complexes (PVCs) in healthy patients are relatively benign and may not require treatment

    c. Ventricular arrhythmias, such as PVCs and ventricular tachycardia, are the most common serious arrhythmias that occur intraoperatively

  2. Causes

    a. Injection of solutions containing cocaine or epinephrine, especially under halothane anesthesia

    b. Carbon dioxide buildup, usually relieved by increased ventilation

    c. Sensitization of the myocardium to catecholamines from halothane and enflurane

    d. Vagal stimulation from surgical manipulation, resulting in sudden bradycardia or asystole

    e. Use of cocaine, which interacts with anesthetics

  3. Treatment by anesthesia team

    a. Identify and correct the underlying cause of the arrhythmia

    b. Prepare for emergency resuscitative measures

  4. Nursing responsibilities

    a. Know the location and operation of the defibrillator and emergency cart because arrhythmia can lead to cardiac arrest

    b. Assist the anesthesia team by readying drug injections and documenting drug administration

    c. Encourage the patient to disclose all drug use preoperatively

## D. Cardiac arrest

  1. General information

    a. Onset is seldom sudden and usually preceded by arrhythmias, hypoxia, or hypotension

   b.  Cardiac arrest is more commonly seen in high-risk patients, those with
       preexisting disease, and those undergoing emergency surgery
2.  Causes
   a.  Hemorrhage and ensuing hypotension
   b.  Cardiac arrhythmias
   c.  Overdose of anesthetic agent
   d.  Sudden hyperkalemia in burn or trauma patients, especially when the
       muscle relaxant succinylcholine is used
   e.  Heart surgery
   f.  Hypoxia
   g.  Surgical manipulation of abdominal viscera or brain
   h.  Malignant hyperthermia (MH)
3.  Treatment by the anesthesia team
   a.  Identify and correct the underlying cause of cardiac arrest
   b.  Institute emergency life support measures
4.  Nursing responsibilities
   a.  Retrieve defibrillator and emergency cart
   b.  Assist the anesthesia team as needed by preparing drugs and I.V.
       infusions
   c.  Notify family members of the situation (with approval of the physician in
       charge), and request spiritual or emotional support persons to be with
       them until outcome is known

E.  **Malignant hyperthermia**
   1.  General information
      a.  MH, a genetically determined hypermetabolic response to certain
          anesthetic agents, is a true emergency and commonly fatal; death can
          occur within minutes of onset unless recognized and treated with
          dantrolene (Dantrium)
      b.  MH does not always occur on anesthesia induction but can occur anytime
          during or after surgery or recur several hours after the initial episode has
          subsided
      c.  Symptoms include tachycardia, increased carbon dioxide production,
          muscle rigidity, arrhythmias, elevated body temperature, unstable blood
          pressure, and cyanosis or mottled skin
      d.  A negative personal or family history does not rule out possible
          occurrence
      e.  Susceptible patients are encouraged to have regional (not general)
          anesthesia
   2.  Causes
      a.  Presence of inherited trait altering the physiologic action of calcium in
          the muscle (MH episode apparently triggers release of excessive amounts
          of calcium from the cells)
      b.  Anesthetic agents, especially the inhalation agent halothane and the
          neuromuscular blocking agent succinylcholine

3. Treatment by anesthesia team
   a. Cool patient by any means possible—packing in ice, iced I.V. infusions, iced saline lavage of body cavities including bladder, stomach, and colon
   b. Inject dantrolene intravenously
   c. Replace anesthesia machine in use with another because triggering agent may still be present in anesthesia circuit
4. Nursing responsibilities
   a. Call for help immediately; several people are needed to obtain ice and pack the patient in it
   b. Obtain iced solutions and ice and assist with packing, infusing, and lavaging the patient
   c. Know where dantrolene is stored, and obtain and begin mixing the solution for I.V. administration as ordered
   d. Retrieve the emergency cart and defibrillator because MH commonly leads to cardiac arrest

F. Volume depletion
   1. General information
      a. A significant loss of circulating blood volume occurs during major surgery but can also develop unexpectedly during routine procedures
      b. Gradual blood loss is better tolerated than sudden blood loss, and a patient who is stable before surgery can better tolerate volume depletion
      c. Jehovah's Witnesses or patients concerned about acquired immunodeficiency syndrome (AIDS) may refuse transfusions to replace lost blood
      d. Anesthesia teams are more cautious about transfusing patients because donor blood may be contaminated with human immunodeficiency virus
   2. Causes
      a. Surgical blood loss
      b. Insufficient replacement with fluids or blood products
      c. Low hematocrit or volume depletion from preoperative trauma or illness
   3. Treatment by anesthesia team
      a. Replace lost blood volume with crystalloid I.V. fluids, such as albumin, plasmanate, and blood or blood products
      b. Administer cardiostimulatory drugs as indicated
   4. Nursing responsibilities
      a. Counsel patients who refuse transfusions preoperatively about potential consequences, even if significant blood loss is not anticipated
      b. Ask the patient to sign the refusal for transfusion form, if available, and place it in the chart
      c. Check availability of compatible blood and have blood typed, crossmatched, and sent to the operating room
      d. Monitor blood lost on discarded sponges, and observe the amount and types of irrigating solutions used
      e. Obtain blood products as ordered, and follow institutional guidelines on patient identification before giving blood products to the anesthesia team

## G. Aspiration pneumonia
1. General information
   a. Aspiration is the introduction of foreign matter into the trachea and lungs; contact with acidic (pH less than 2.5) stomach contents results in inflammation and direct injury to airway passages, possibly leading to fatal pneumonia
   b. General anesthesia, including mask anesthesia, obtunds the protective gag and swallowing reflexes, causing aspiration in some patients
2. Causes
   a. Ingestion of food or drink less than 8 hours before surgery
   b. Catecholamine release and anxiety from trauma
   c. Increased intragastric pressure (obstetric patients)
   d. Esophageal reflux
3. Prevention
   a. Use cuffed endotracheal tube that seals off lungs from stomach contents
   b. Perform preoperative aspiration prophylaxis — orally administer a clear nonparticulate antacid, parenterally administer a histamine receptor-blocking drug, and orally or parentally administer metoclopramide (Reclomide) to increase stomach emptying
   c. Execute rapid-sequence (or "crash") induction in a patient at risk, consisting of preoxygenation for 5 minutes, cricoid pressure on induction and until the endotracheal tube cuff is inflated, and rapid intubation without mask ventilation; extubate the patient when he is awake and swallowing and gag reflexes are intact
4. Treatment by anesthesia team
   a. Stop surgery to evaluate the patient if aspiration occurs
   b. Obtain chest X-ray and blood gas analysis
   c. Administer steroids and antibiotics
   d. Request pulmonary consultation
5. Nursing responsibilities
   a. Explain the importance of adhering to nothing-by-mouth (NPO) orders, and verify NPO status before taking the patient to the surgical suite
   b. Learn the proper method of applying cricoid pressure
   c. Assist in securing the airway by applying cricoid pressure, as indicated, and do not release this pressure until instructed by the anesthesia team

## Points to Remember

Intraoperative complications are rare but may be swift and fatal.

The perioperative nurse's actions have a significant impact on the outcome of the emergency.

Malignant hyperthermia is an infrequent but serious complication that may end in death.

Patients must be evaluated for compliance with NPO orders before being taken to the surgical suite.

Every perioperative nurse should know the location of the defibrillator, emergency cart, tracheotomy tray, dantrolene, and iced solutions before starting a case.

## Glossary

**Aspiration pneumonia** — injury to lungs and bronchioles from contact with acid stomach contents, causing inflammation and direct harm to airway passages

**Cricothyrotomy** — procedure in which the surgeon makes a small vertical incision into the larynx to open a patient's airway

**Malignant hyperthermia** — genetically determined and commonly fatal hypermetabolic response to the administration of certain anesthetic agents

**Premature ventricular complex** — cardiac arrhythmia characterized by a ventricular beat that precedes the expected electrical impulse; appears on an electrocardiogram as an early, wide QRS complex without a preceding P wave

**Temporomandibular joint** — gliding, hingelike joint that connects the mandible to the temporal bone

# Postoperative Nursing

**Learning Objectives**

After studying this section, the reader should be able to:

• Describe key postoperative assessments.

• List necessary postoperative equipment and supplies.

• Cite potential complications of recovery from general anesthesia.

• Discuss nursing responsibilities relevant to care of a patient recovering from general, regional, or local anesthesia.

## XI. Postoperative Nursing

### A. Introduction

1. The postoperative phase begins with admission of the patient to the postanesthesia care unit (PACU) and ends when surgery-related nursing care is no longer required
2. A major postoperative task is termination of the anesthetic, which is performed gradually
3. Responsibility for postoperative patient care is shared by the following:
   a. Anesthesia team (until care is assumed by a PACU nurse)
   b. PACU nurse (while the patient recovers from anesthesia)
   c. Postoperative nurse (when the patient is transferred to a nursing unit)
4. The goal of postoperative nursing is to facilitate recovery through continuous and careful patient monitoring while preserving and respecting patient dignity (see Appendix C, Nursing Process Applied to the Postoperative Phase)
5. Constant vigilance is essential because serious complications can lead to aspiration, hypoxia, cardiac arrest, brain damage, and death
6. Equipment needed at the patient's bedside in the PACU includes:
   a. Oxygen source
   b. Oxygen face mask and delivery system adapted for endotracheal tube
   c. Nasal and oral airways
   d. Suction
   e. Syringes and needles
7. Equipment needed at the patient's bedside in the nursing unit includes:
   a. Oxygen source
   b. Suction
   c. Dressings and wound care supplies, such as tape and solutions
   d. Items specific to the patient's condition and surgery, such as nasogastric tubes and drainage collection containers
8. Equipment that should be readily available in the PACU and nursing unit includes:
   a. Manual resuscitation bag
   b. Ventilator
   c. Emergency drugs
   d. Defibrillator
   e. Laryngoscopes and endotracheal tubes
9. Postoperative assessments and interventions focus on:
   a. Respiratory status — airway patency; rate, depth, and character of respirations
   b. Circulatory status — vital signs, heart rate and rhythm, pulse rate, skin and mucous membrane color
   c. Temperature — shivering, diaphoresis
   d. Neurologic status — level of consciousness, reflexes, muscle strength, sensory perception
   e. Skin integrity — wound site, dressings, drainage

f. Urinary function—presence of drainage tubes; amount, color, and characteristics of urine
g. Gastrointestinal function—presence and character of bowel sounds, passage of flatus or stool, nausea, presence of decompression tubes (such as nasogastric tubes)
h. Fluid and electrolyte balance—hydration status, intake and output, diagnostic studies, fluid replacements and drainage
i. Comfort—signs and symptoms of pain, analgesics administered intraoperatively

**B. Patient recovering from general anesthesia**
1. General information
   a. A patient recovering from general anesthesia is at risk for complications
   b. On arriving in the PACU, a patient is assessed for airway patency, vital signs, level of consciousness, skin color, patency of drains, status of I.V. infusions and insertion sites, appearance of surgical site and dressings, and need for monitoring equipment, such as electrocardiograph and pulse oximeter
2. Complications
   a. Laryngospasm from airway irritation and sudden closure of vocal cords, heralded by noisy respirations, cyanosis, chest retractions, and increased abdominal movement
   b. Hypoxia from airway obstruction, laryngospasm, hypoventilation, or accumulation of secretions
   c. Hypotension from residual effects of anesthetic agents, unreplenished surgical blood loss, and movement
   d. Hypertension from hypercapnia and hypoxia, pain, and hypothermia
   e. Malignant hyperthermia
   f. Emergence delirium characterized by excitement, thrashing, and incoherent or irrational speech
   g. Uncontrolled pain leading to tachycardia, hypertension, and cardiovascular collapse
3. Nursing responsibilities
   a. Assess the patient's airway patency and adequacy of respirations immediately on admission, and communicate any concerns to the anesthesia team
   b. Check the patient's blood pressure, and notify the anesthesia team of hypotension or hypertension
   c. Administer oxygen, as ordered, through the airway, using a face mask or endotracheal tube connector
   d. Apply the face mask carefully; a semiconscious or unconscious patient has inadequate corneal reflexes and may sustain corneal abrasions if the mask or straps touch the eyes

e.  Administer oxygen by positive pressure, using a manual resuscitation bag and mask; lift the jaw to open the airway; and place the patient in a sitting position when possible to relieve laryngospasm

f.  Anticipate administration of succinylcholine (relaxes vocal cord muscles) by the anesthesia team and manual ventilation until neuromuscular function returns

g.  Position an unconscious patient on his side to reduce possible airway obstruction by the tongue and to prevent aspiration; elevate the head of the bed to facilitate breathing

h.  Obtain an order for and administer pain medications as indicated

i.  To relieve nausea, apply a cool, damp washcloth to the patient's face and neck, administer antiemetics as ordered, and minimize position changes

j.  Follow institutional guidelines for extubation

k.  Limit bedside conversation and do not discuss prognosis because the patient can hear but may misinterpret what is said

l.  Apply warm blankets or heat lamps as necessary for a hypothermic or shivering patient

m.  If the patient must be intubated and mechanically ventilated, consider requesting an order for a benzodiazepine to minimize recall of this unpleasant experience

n.  Pull drapes and provide privacy when examining the patient or offering a bedpan, but do not leave drapes pulled around a semiconscious or unconscious patient; observation is essential to early detection of respiratory obstruction, cyanosis, and apnea

o.  Put side rails up to prevent falls, and assist the patient in leaving the bed to prevent orthostatic hypotension

p.  Do not offer water or ice chips until ordered and the patient is fully awake and does not need to return to surgery

## C.  Patient recovering from local or regional anesthesia

1.  General information

a.  The patient has usually received sedatives that may alter the sensorium and also has difficulty controlling movement of limbs affected by the anesthetic

b.  Following safety precautions can help minimize the risk of injury to the patient

2.  Complications

a.  The risk of most complications has passed by the time a patient is admitted to the PACU

b.  Vigilance is still necessary because sedatives and narcotics may have been administered, and surgical complications can occur

3. Nursing responsibilities
   a. Assess the patient's condition, including cardiopulmonary status, level of consciousness, and sensory and motor function
   b. Reassure a patient concerned about inability to move extremities, and discuss progression of return of function
   c. Align affected extremities correctly and pad pressure points; residual anesthetic effects may prevent the patient from complaining of discomfort
   d. Raise side rails to prevent falls, and assist the patient in getting out of bed because motor control may be poor

## Points to Remember

Termination of an anesthetic is a gradual process.

The PACU nurse assumes much responsibility for the patient recovering from anesthesia.

Constant vigilance is essential while a patient recovers from anesthesia; serious complications can lead to aspiration, hypoxia, cardiac arrest, brain damage, and death.

An unconscious patient must never be left unattended.

## Glossary

**Emergence** — time from discontinuation of anesthetic to appropriate patient response to commands

**Emergence delirium** — excitement, thrashing, and incoherent speech as patient recovers from general anesthesia

**Hypoventilation** — ventilation insufficient in rate or depth to maintain adequate oxygen in the blood and eliminate carbon dioxide

**Hypoxia** — insufficient oxygen in the blood

**Laryngospasm** — closure of vocal cords, usually in response to painful stimulus or airway irritation

# Ambulatory Surgery

**Learning Objectives**

After studying this section, the reader should be able to:

● Define ambulatory surgery and list its advantages.

● Discuss the importance of documentation and patient teaching.

● Describe nursing responsibilities relevant to care of a patient undergoing ambulatory surgery.

# XII. Ambulatory Surgery

## A. Introduction

1. Refers to surgery in which the patient is admitted and discharged on the same day (also called one-day, outpatient, same-day, or short-stay surgery)
2. Has become increasingly prevalent in recent years because of:
   a. Demands for cost containment and cost effectiveness
   b. Technologic advances in equipment and medication
   c. Advantages of early ambulation, home convalescence, and early return to presurgical functioning
   d. Overall satisfaction of all parties
3. Is performed in many settings, including hospital-affiliated centers, independent free-standing facilities, and physicians' offices
4. Has several advantages:
   a. Reduced patient and third-party cost
   b. Rapid return to familiar, less stressful environment
   c. Decreased period of patient dependency
   d. Elimination of psychological trauma of hospitalization
   e. Reduced risk of nosocomial infections
   f. More efficient use of hospital bed space
   g. More personalized and individualized patient care
5. Requires nursing care similar to that for inpatient surgery—standards, principles, and procedures are the same (although assessments, time allotments, teaching, and follow-up may vary)
6. Necessitates efficient, well-documented nursing care because interaction between patient and perioperative team may occur in only a few hours

## B. Preoperative phase

1. General information
   a. Patients selected for ambulatory surgery usually meet P1 or P2 criteria of the American Society of Anesthesiologists' status classification (see *Physical status classification for anesthesia classification* on page 31 in Section IV for more information)
   b. Preadmission testing (diagnostic studies and preanesthesia patient evaluation) is ideally performed days in advance but may be done on the morning of surgery
   c. Patients usually receive written instructions about perioperative events, including preoperative preparation and discharge procedures, when visiting the surgeon or reporting for preadmission testing
   d. The preoperative nurse usually calls the patient on the day before surgery to review written instructions, confirm the time to report to the facility, and request that someone accompany the patient home after discharge
   e. Family members are usually allowed to stay with the patient until transfer to the operating room

  f. A patient may walk to the operating room or be transported in a wheelchair, reclining chair, or stretcher, depending on the patient's abilities, medications given, and the facility's policies

  g. Accurate, clear, and thorough communication, documentation, and patient teaching are essential to successful ambulatory surgery

 2. Nursing responsibilities

  a. Confirm the date and time of preadmission testing, and arrange to meet the patient to explain preoperative events and orient him to the facility

  b. Review written instructions or brochures given to the patient, emphasizing preoperative restrictions and the need for a family member or friend to accompany the patient home

  c. Call the patient the day before surgery to reinforce written instructions

  d. Apply a patient identification band on the day of surgery, and help the patient secure any valuables and change into appropriate surgical attire

  e. Assess the patient's physical and psychosocial status

  f. Verify that the patient's chart contains all necessary information (diagnostic tests, signed informed consent documents, preanesthesia evaluation)

  g. Administer preoperative medications as ordered, and offer comfort measures (extra blankets or pillows) and diversions (television or music) to alleviate patient anxiety

  h. Explain the procedure to the patient and family

  i. To promote continuity of care, document all preoperative assessments, interventions, teaching, and events in the patient's record, and assist with patient transfer to the operating room

## C. Intraoperative phase

 1. General information

  a. Many patients undergo local or regional anesthesia

  b. If general anesthesia is administered, surgery is scheduled early in the day to allow the patient adequate time to recover

 2. Nursing responsibilities

  a. Follow the same principles, procedures, and techniques used for inpatient surgery

  b. Document all intraoperative events

## D. Postoperative phase

 1. General information

  a. Ambulatory surgery usually involves a rapid recovery

  b. Patient care principles are similar to those of inpatient surgery

  c. Discharge criteria include stable vital signs; presence of gag reflex; ability to walk, void, and tolerate fluids; normal level of consciousness; and little if any bleeding, drainage, or pain

  d. Written discharge instructions are usually given to the patient and family members

2. Nursing responsibilities
   a. Assess the patient's overall status, check for presence of gag reflex, and offer fluids if appropriate
   b. Assist the patient in using a bedpan, getting out of bed, standing, or walking to the bathroom, and encourage progressive ambulation
   c. Administer medication as ordered for pain, nausea, or vomiting
   d. Promote patient comfort and relaxation, and allow family members to stay with the patient
   e. Provide written and oral discharge instructions, including any restrictions and medical follow-up, and make a follow-up telephone call to evaluate the patient's status
   f. Document all events in the patient's record
   g. Accompany the patient to the facility's exit, and discharge him to the care of a responsible family member or friend

## Points to Remember

Nursing standards, principles, and procedures for ambulatory surgery are the same as those for inpatient surgery.

Documentation, communication, and patient teaching are essential components of perioperative nursing for ambulatory surgery.

Patient assessment, including diagnostic tests and preanesthesia evaluation, are usually performed days in advance of surgery.

A responsible family member or friend must accompany the patient home.

## Glossary

**Discharge instructions** — information given to the patient about necessary home care

**Nosocomial infection** — infection acquired in a hospital

**Preadmission testing** — diagnostic procedures and tests done in advance of surgery

# Legal Considerations

**Learning Objectives**

After studying this section, the reader should be able to:

- List three legal doctrines that apply to perioperative nursing.

- Identify at least five possible sources of legal action against a perioperative nurse.

- Discuss nursing actions that can minimize the risk of a lawsuit.

## XIII. Legal Considerations

### A. Introduction

1. The legal duty of a perioperative nurse is to provide reasonable and prudent care, ensure patient safety, and prevent patient injury
2. Perioperative nurses practice in many settings, including operating rooms, specialized procedure rooms, one-day surgery areas, and outpatient surgical facilities
3. Perioperative nursing standards emphasize patient safety because of the inherent danger and sophisticated nature of surgical equipment and procedures
4. Three major legal doctrines cover problems associated with perioperative injuries
   a. According to the *borrowed servant* doctrine, nurses working in the operating room are both hospital employees and under the direction of the surgeon; thus, liability for negligence lies with the nurse, hospital, and surgeon
   b. Based on the legal concept of *res ipsa loquitur* ("the thing speaks for itself"), injuries to an anesthetized (usually unconscious) patient could have been caused only by the negligence of the surgical team; thus, the burden of proof is on the defendants rather than the plaintiff
   c. Perioperative nurses are liable for their own negligent acts under the doctrine of *respondeat superior,* even if the hospital and surgeon are also liable
5. A perioperative nurse cannot deny responsibility for a harmful act or inaction on the grounds that someone else was also responsible

### B. Sources of legal action

1. General information
   a. A surgical patient is completely dependent on those caring for him
   b. Surgery inherently involves intrusive and potentially destructive actions by health care professionals
   c. A heavily sedated or unconscious patient cannot feel pain or take actions to prevent further infliction of injury
   d. Equipment that is defective or misused can result in patient injury
   e. Legal action against a perioperative nurse usually involves issues of patient safety
2. Failure to obtain informed consent
   a. Perioperative nurses must ensure that a surgeon has obtained the patient's informed consent before surgery and must document this in the patient's record
   b. Failure to obtain informed consent before surgery violates the patient's right to self-determination and can lead to illegal, fraudulent, or contraindicated procedures

3. Retained foreign objects
   a. Retained foreign objects (such as sponges or needles) fall under the *res ipsa loquitur* doctrine and constitute the most common type of negligence involving perioperative nurses
   b. The statute of limitations varies because patients do not always know immediately after surgery that a foreign object has been retained
4. Abandonment
   a. Abandonment occurs when a health care professional ends a relationship with a patient without the patient's consent (for example, when a nurse leaves a patient unattended)
   b. Defending against the charge of abandonment is especially difficult for a perioperative nurse because an anesthetized patient cannot legally provide consent
5. Scope of practice violations
   a. A nurse cannot legally perform duties considered outside the scope of nursing practice
   b. Malpractice insurance policies generally do not cover nurses who function in this capacity
6. Safety violations
   a. Failure to monitor a patient recovering from anesthesia is a common charge brought against perioperative nurses, particularly those in the postanesthesia care unit (PACU)
   b. Improper positioning of a patient and use of defective equipment produce the most common perioperative injuries, such as peroneal nerve paralysis and burns
   c. Inaccurate patient identification can lead to an assault charge if the patient undergoes surgery for which he was not scheduled
7. Wrongful death
   a. Wrongful death lawsuits have been brought against PACU nurses
   b. Most such cases have involved an inexperienced nurse who failed to detect hypoxia or a lethal arrhythmia or who discharged a patient to a room in the nursing unit before the patient was fully awake

## C. Implications for perioperative nurses

1. Adhering to established safety procedures helps prevent injuries to the patient, thus minimizing the risk of a lawsuit
2. Perioperative nurses must ensure that informed consent has been obtained and documented
3. Careful counting of sponges, needles, and other equipment during surgery is essential to prevent a foreign object from being retained in a patient's body
4. An unconscious patient should never be left unattended; other patients may be left unattended only when absolutely necessary to their care (for example, to retrieve emergency medications)

5. A perioperative nurse working as first surgical assistant is held to the standards of care for that profession and, in some states, may lose her nursing license
6. Complete and accurate documentation helps prevent injury and serves as a record of safety measures taken, thus enabling a nurse to refute a negligence charge
7. Perioperative nurses should be involved in the development of institutional safety procedures, policies, and precautions

## Points to Remember

All nurses are legally liable to provide reasonable and prudent care.

The intrusive and potentially destructive nature of surgery and the inability of patients to protect themselves place additional liability on perioperative nurses.

Legal action against perioperative nurses commonly involves failure to check for informed consent, retention of foreign objects, improper patient positioning, or use of defective equipment.

The best defense against legal action is to avoid injury by ensuring patient safety.

## Glossary

**Defendant** — person against whom a lawsuit is brought because of alleged wrongdoing

**Liability** — legal obligation or responsibility

**Plaintiff** — person who initiates a lawsuit

**Res ipsa loquitur** — legal concept that allows a plaintiff (patient) to sue for negligence based on circumstantial evidence, thereby shifting the burden of proof to the defendant (surgical team)

# Appendices

## Appendix A

### NURSING PROCESS APPLIED TO THE PREOPERATIVE PHASE

The preoperative nurse uses the nursing process when caring for a surgical patient. The following chart identifies each step of the nursing process and relevant nursing responsibilities.

| STEP | NURSING RESPONSIBILITIES |
|---|---|
| Assessment | • Obtain a nursing history from the patient (reason for admission, personal and family history of illnesses, previous and current medications).<br>• Perform a physical assessment, including a review of systems, nutritional status, and height and weight measurements.<br>• Determine the patient's level of understanding about the planned surgery.<br>• Identify risk factors that may interfere with surgery (such as advanced age, obesity, history of cardiac problems, or malnutrition).<br>• Assess the patient's psychosocial status, including anxiety level and availability of family members and friends for emotional support. |
| Diagnosis | • Analyze assessment information to determine appropriate nursing diagnostic categories; common ones include:<br>—Anxiety<br>—Knowledge deficit<br>—Fear<br>—Self-esteem disturbance<br>—Pain<br>—Altered role performance<br>—Altered nutrition: Less than body requirements |
| Planning | • Develop patient-centered goals based on identified nursing diagnoses.<br>• Anticipate potential risk factors and inform the physician. |
| Implementation | • Orient the patient to the surgical unit.<br>• Explain the purpose of diagnostic tests, the preanesthesia evaluation, and preoperative medications.<br>• Instruct the patient on all aspects of planned surgical events.<br>• Teach the patient postoperative exercises (such as coughing, deep breathing, isometric leg exercises) that can help prevent complications and facilitate recovery.<br>• Review the importance of dietary restrictions, such as nothing-by-mouth orders.<br>• Discuss the possible need for I.V. lines or nasogastric tubes, and explain their benefits.<br>• Allow the patient to express concerns and fears about the |

**NURSING PROCESS APPLIED TO THE PREOPERATIVE PHASE** *continued*

| STEP | NURSING RESPONSIBILITIES |
|---|---|
| Implementation *continued* | surgery, and offer emotional support and guidance to the patient and family.<br>• Witness the patient's signature to the informed consent.<br>• Administer sedatives as prescribed.<br>• Carry out preoperative skin preparation as ordered.<br>• Ensure that all necessary information is documented on the patient's record.<br>• Complete the preoperative checklist.<br>• Premedicate the patient as ordered.<br>• Inform the patient of safety precautions to take once medication has been administered.<br>• Assist in transferring the patient from the hospital bed to the stretcher.<br>• Ensure that the patient's identification band is in place. |
| Evaluation | • Have the patient repeat instructions given and demonstrate techniques taught to determine the effectiveness of your teaching.<br>• Evaluate the patient's progress in meeting predetermined goals.<br>• Revise the care plan if goals have not been achieved or only partially met. |

# Appendix B

## NURSING PROCESS APPLIED TO THE INTRAOPERATIVE PHASE

The circulating and scrub nurses use the nursing process when caring for a patient intraoperatively. The following chart identifies each step of the nursing process and relevant nursing responsibilities.

| STEP | NURSING RESPONSIBILITIES |
|---|---|
| Assessment | • Review the patient's record when he arrives in the preoperative holding area.<br>• Check the patient's identification band to ensure that the correct patient has arrived.<br>• Review the preoperative checklist, and notify the surgeon of any problems or changes.<br>• Verify that the patient's signed consent form is included in the chart.<br>• Assess the patient's overall condition, including level of consciousness and anxiety level.<br>• Assess the planned operation site for condition and preoperative preparation, such as shaving. |
| Diagnosis | • Analyze assessment information to determine appropriate nursing diagnostic categories; common ones include:<br>—Anxiety<br>—Impaired verbal communication<br>—Fear<br>—Potential for injury<br>—Knowledge deficit<br>—Impaired skin integrity<br>—Altered tissue perfusion<br>—Potential for aspiration<br>—Ineffective breathing pattern<br>—Fluid volume deficit<br>—Fluid volume overload<br>—Impaired gas exchange |
| Planning | • Develop patient-centered goals based on identified nursing diagnoses.<br>• Anticipate needed equipment and supplies, and prepare the operating room.<br>• Check the surgeon's preference card for information about sutures, instruments, and other supplies needed for surgery.<br>• Identify aspects of the operating room that may interfere with the patient's well-being, such as an excessively cool temperature. |
| Implementation | • Perform scrub procedures according to institutional policy; dress in the appropriate surgical attire, including gown, gloves, shoe covers, and mask.<br>• Set up the operating room with the appropriate equipment and supplies for the type of surgery planned.<br>• When the patient enters the operating room, recheck the patient's identification band.<br>• Position the patient appropriately for surgery. |

## NURSING PROCESS APPLIED TO THE INTRAOPERATIVE PHASE *continued*

| STEP | NURSING RESPONSIBILITIES |
|------|--------------------------|
| Implementation *continued* | • Assist the anesthesia team as necessary.<br>• Assist the surgeon as necessary (scrub nurse).<br>• Help obtain additional supplies and equipment (circulating nurse).<br>• Inform the surgeon or the anesthesia team of changes in the patient's condition.<br>• Perform counts on surgical instruments and supplies.<br>• Maintain aseptic technique.<br>• Monitor the patient's physiologic status.<br>• Document all observations and actions on the patient's record.<br>• Provide emotional support when the patient is recovering from anesthesia.<br>• Assist in transferring the patient from the operating room to the postanesthesia care unit.<br>• Act as a patient advocate by maintaining the patient's privacy and providing for his safety. |
| Evaluation | • Determine whether surgery went as planned.<br>• Identify modifications to the postoperative plan of care warranted by the surgical outcome. |

# Appendix C

## NURSING PROCESS APPLIED TO THE POSTOPERATIVE PHASE

The postanesthesia care unit (PACU) nurse and the postoperative nurse use the nursing process when caring for a patient postoperatively. The following chart identifies each step of the nursing process and relevant nursing responsibilities.

| STEP | NURSING RESPONSIBILITIES |
|---|---|
| Assessment | *Immediately*<br>• Prepare the PACU for the patient's arrival.<br>• Obtain reports from the anesthesia team, surgeon, and intraoperative nurses.<br>• Review the patient's record for the type of surgery performed and preoperative and intraoperative status.<br>• Assess the patient's overall condition, particularly respiratory and circulatory functioning.<br>*Upon return to the nursing unit*<br>• Prepare the patient's bed on the nursing unit.<br>• Obtain a report from the PACU nurse about the patient's recovery and status.<br>• Check the surgeon's postoperative orders. |
| Diagnosis | • Analyze assessment information to determine appropriate nursing diagnostic categories; common ones include:<br>— Pain<br>— Impaired skin integrity<br>— Ineffective airway clearance<br>— Sensory-perceptual alterations<br>— Impaired physical mobility<br>— Potential for altered body temperature<br>— Anxiety<br>— Potential for aspiration<br>— Potential for injury |
| Planning | • Anticipate the need for equipment and supplies, and arrange them at the patient's bedside.<br>• Develop patient-centered goals based on identified nursing diagnoses. |
| Implementation | *Immediately*<br>• Ensure that all necessary equipment is available.<br>• Perform a review of body systems, including airway, vital signs, and level of consciousness.<br>• Turn the patient on his side to prevent aspiration, and suction as necessary.<br>• Inspect drainage tubes for the type, amount, and character of drainage; irrigate tubes, if ordered.<br>• Inspect I.V. infusions and regulate flow rates, as needed.<br>• Monitor skin color and capillary refill time.<br>• Inspect the wound and dressings for drainage or bleeding.<br>• Monitor the patient's fluid intake and output.<br>• Use a moist washcloth or swabsticks to relieve mouth dryness. |

**NURSING PROCESS APPLIED TO THE POSTOPERATIVE PHASE** *continued*

| STEP | NURSING RESPONSIBILITIES |
| --- | --- |
| Implementation *continued* | • Orient the patient to his surroundings and explain what is happening.<br>• Offer pain medication, if ordered.<br>• Document all actions and observations on the patient's record.<br>*Upon return to the nursing unit*<br>• Ensure that all necessary equipment is available.<br>• Place the bed in a high position to facilitate patient transfer from stretcher to bed.<br>• Perform a review of body systems, including airway, vital signs, and level of consciousness.<br>• Position the patient on his side, using pillows for support.<br>• Monitor skin color and temperature.<br>• Inspect the wound site and dressings for bleeding or drainage. Note the amount, type, and character of drainage.<br>• Check I.V. fluids and adjust flow rates, as ordered.<br>• Palpate the patient's abdomen, if not contraindicated, for bladder distention; if an indwelling urinary catheter is present, make sure it is patent and draining; offer a bedpan or urinal if no catheter is present.<br>• Measure the patient's fluid intake and output.<br>• Change the patient's position every 2 hours, maintaining correct body alignment.<br>• Monitor for complaints of nausea and vomiting.<br>• Medicate as ordered for pain or nausea.<br>• Speak with the patient and family about the patient's status and expectations.<br>• Explain the purpose of equipment and interventions.<br>• Encourage early and progressive ambulation. Assist the patient in getting out of bed to prevent orthostatic hypotension.<br>• Inform the patient of dietary restrictions, such as nothing-by-mouth or clear liquid orders.<br>• Notify the physician of any changes in the patient's condition.<br>• Encourage coughing and deep-breathing exercises and incentive spirometry.<br>• Gradually increase the patient's participation in self-care.<br>• Discuss discharge plans with the patient and family; assist with any referrals to outside agencies or personnel.<br>• Document all actions and observations in the patient's record. |
| Evaluation | • Compare the patient's progress with predetermined goals, and evaluate the need for changes to the care plan.<br>• Ask the patient to demonstrate skills taught and to repeat instructions given.<br>• Confirm that the patient or a family member can adequately care for the patient after discharge. |

# Index

i refers to an illustration; t refers to a table.

i refers to an illustration; t refers to a table.